Caring for Health

SUSAN PROCTER

First published 2000 by
MACMILLAN PRESS LTD
Houndmills, Basingstoke, Hampshire RG21 6XS
and London
Companies and representatives
throughout the world

ISBN 0–333–62248–0 paperback

A catalogue record for this book is available
from the British Library.

This book is printed on paper suitable for recycling and
made from fully managed and sustained forest sources.

10 9   8   7   6   5   4   3   2   1
09 08 07 06 05 04 03 02 01 00

Editing and origination by
Aardvark Editorial, Mendham, Suffolk

Printed in Malaysia

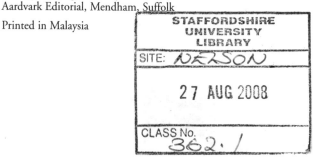

To my sons
Daniel and Richard

Contents

List of Figures, Tables and Vignettes

Figures

Tables

Vignettes

Acknowledgements

There are two people without whom this book would not have been written. The first to whom I am indebted is Jo Campling, who in the dim and distant past first approached me with the idea of writing a book something like the one produced here, and who has stood by me unfailingly throughout the highs and lows of its production. The second person is Richenda Milton-Thompson, my publisher, who has provided continued support and encouragement throughout the long gestation period of the book.

I am also indebted to my colleagues at the University of Northumbria – Jan Reed, Charlotte Clarke, Bill Watson, Sue Croom, Vera Swallow to name but a few whose lively ideas and debates, difficult to attribute individually, are woven into the fabric of the book. Thanks must also go to Anne Hanson for her skill and patience in editing and proofing the final manuscript.

Finally, I must thank my family for their unfailing support and encouragement and for not complaining about my prolonged absences during the writing of this book.

Chapter 1

Introduction

This book is about nursing and health. It sets out to demarcate the specific contribution that nurses make to health and in so doing highlights the importance of caring processes to health care outcomes.

The book identifies the problems for health created by a failure in caring processes, regardless of whether the failure occurs in public institutions such as hospitals, community care services or residential care; in semi-institutional settings such as foster care or nurseries, or with childminders or nannies; or privately within families. Caring is a universal attribute necessary for health and human survival and cannot be claimed by any one professional group. Nursing is, however, developing a rigorous and systematic body of knowledge about caring processes, in particular those caring processes associated with physical care, intimacy, frailty, vulnerability, dependency, inter-dependency, growth and autonomy. In developing this knowledge base, nursing focuses particularly on the health outcomes embedded in the daily routines through which individuals, families and paid carers manage activities of living (for example eating, sleeping, leisure, exercise and socialising) over the 24-hour period. Each of these activities of living is inextricably linked to health, and the processes and routines by which individuals, families and paid carers manage these activities, over the 24-hour period, influence the ongoing and long-term health status of the individual or recipient of care.

Nursing knowledge about caring processes is derived from the practice of nursing and from the investment in nursing arising from the educational opportunities afforded nurses internationally as part of their academic and professional development. Nursing is, therefore, privileged to be able to develop a unique body of knowledge about caring processes, which will inform not only the profession of nursing, but also the work of carers wherever they are located and however they are supported or funded. The importance of caring processes for health promotion and maintenance means that nursing has a critical academic and practice role to play in shaping the understanding of the adverse consequences of a failure to care on health outcomes. This role includes increasing knowledge about the support required to prevent such failures in care.

Ann Oakley (1996) in her biography of the lives of her parents, pays tribute to the radicalism that characterised her father, Richard Titmuss', work. The work of Richard Titmuss and his colleagues laid down the foundation for welfare reform across Europe following the Second World War. As Ann Oakley states:

> Richard Titmuss' work represented radicalism, of a kind. It was informed by a passionate belief that human beings could only fulfil their potential in a society that offered equality for all. Underpinning his vision was a profound moral sense that an equal society would also be one based on caring and altruism; a 'good' society could not be a self-serving one, in which everyone looked after their own interests and ignored those of others. (Oakley, 1996, p. 4)

However, as Ann Oakley points out, the analysis given by Titmuss of power relations in social institutions, in tax reform and in health and education policy was profoundly blind to the deep fissure created by the different social experiences of men and women. Oakley suggests that, to Titmuss, gendered experiences were not about power but were raised above politics and located in the private sphere of domesticity. The experiences of women and the contributions of women to domestic life were considered sacred and not to be contaminated by the grubbiness of everyday politics.

As a result of this blindness to gendered experiences, post-war policies failed to recognise the impact of politics on the lives, happiness, fortunes and misery of women and the people they care for. The central concern to segregate the public and private spheres of people's lives, which embodied post-war radicalism in Europe, provides a powerful explanation of why the 'social transformatory vision' of the post-war era 'has fizzled out to become a damp squid of post-modern, post-welfarism – a story of increasing misery, acquisitiveness and social inequality' (Oakley, 1996, p. 6).

This book argues that nursing has been marginalised in health care in the UK because, in establishing the National Health Service (NHS), the radical principles that underpinned the vision of social reformers like

Titmuss became the founding principles of the NHS, the gender blindness of social policy transferred into the NHS. The work of nurses, like the work of women in the domestic arena, was considered sacred and above the daily politics of health care provision. Today, the health service is floundering because it is able to recognise neither the inequality that gender blindness has created for the workforce of the NHS, nor the centrality of the work undertaken by nurses in promoting health and curbing avarice and the abuse of medical technology.

The 1980s and 90s were characterised by a literature that testified to the difficulties confronting nursing and the seemingly dysfunctional behaviour of nurses in addressing some of these difficulties (White, 1985; Mackay, 1989; Davies, 1992). Nurses were struggling to gain a political voice in a world that demanded equality with men and failed to acknowledge the quite distinctive experiences and contribution of women and nurses to sustaining and nurturing health.

That tide appears to be changing, and this book contributes to that change. It does not apologise for nursing; it does not criticise nurses; it does not view nursing as a problem. Instead, it seeks to identify the strengths of nursing. It locates the roots of nursing in the caring work attributed to women in the domestic arena. It seeks to identify the health gains that could accrue from developing a shared understanding of health work that breaches the public/private sphere, reintroducing a radicalism that was absent when the NHS was established.

In developing the analysis of nursing and caring work, the book does not seek to devalue the caring contribution that men can and do make in the domestic arena, in nursing and in health and social care. Rather, it recognises the 'clash of masculinities' identified by Davies (1995), who suggests that 'Men may also resist the existing forms of the masculine vision; in doing so they may create a clash of masculinities, or ally with women in a bid for change' (p. 185). Similarly, Robinson (1989) has called for a reconsideration of the gendered assumptions concerning the division of caring labour and a recognition of caring behaviours wherever they occur, regardless of the gender of the person performing them.

This book is also about health. The debates about gender, caring and nursing have to date been confined to a discussion about gendered power relations and the structure of bureaucracies and professions that undermine female experiences, career paths and academic and practice-based interests. This book provides an analysis of the evidence underpinning the maintenance and promotion of health. It highlights how caring work, wherever it is located and regardless of who carries it out, is increasingly being recognised as fundamental to health. It argues that, in the light of this evidence, the marginalisation of caring from health and social care institutions and policy debates becomes increasingly difficult to sustain. If health care institutions do not themselves wish to become marginalised from health, they need to recognise, research, value and reward caring, as only through an acknowledgement of the power of caring in promoting health will the relevance of health *care* institutions to the challenges of the new millennium be maintained.

Chapter 2 provides a description of a range of contemporary theoretical definitions of health. It divides these definitions of health into two categories: selective definitions of health and universal definitions of health. It illustrates how selective definitions of health dominate our understanding of health care provision and constrain the practice of health care professionals, limiting the impact that health care professionals and institutions are able to make to sustain health.

Chapter 3 provides an overview of contemporary demographic and epidemiological trends in wealthy, industrialised countries. It highlights the improvements in life expectancy experienced in most of these countries and cites evidence indicating that these improvements derive from an increasing access to wealth. There is evidence, however, that inequalities in the distribution of wealth within a given society are mirrored in inequalities in health. The chapter also indicates how contemporary disease patterns in industrialised countries are characterised by degenerative diseases that tend to be chronic rather than acute. Medical intervention has improved symptom control and increased life expectancy, but has as yet not been able to reduce disability-free life years. Increasingly wealthy industrialised societies are faced with an ageing population for whom the last few years of life are characterised by chronic degenerative disease processes.

Chapter 3 also reviews the evidence on the efficacy of medical technology in ameliorating disease processes. The evidence indicates an anticipated growth in both the range and the cost of medical technology, but very little evidence to suggest that the costs are matched by equal improvements in health gain. The chapter concludes by arguing that, in the face of an ageing population in whom degenerative diseases predominate, services that promote independence and address the psychological, social and emotional problems that arise when dealing with this type of illness will be fundamental in mediating the demand for health technology.

Chapters 2 and 3 are both about health; Chapter 4 is about care. It provides a brief description of the main features of the philosophical and theoretical literature on care. It recognises that, from a philosophical perspective, caring is frequently defined as a universal and innate human trait. The practice of caring can take a number of forms, one of which relates to the physical and tending aspects of caring. This form of caring is frequently defined as 'women's work' and is located in family care. A range of paid carers are available to substitute for family care, including nurses, residential care workers, nannies, foster parents, childminders and nursery nurses. They are, however, expected to undertake their work unobtrusively and to conform to established family patterns of care. Within contemporary social policy literature, family care is viewed as sacrosanct, and social policy analysts are concerned to ensure that social policies do not interfere with family care or undermine the caring role of the family. This is set against a range of literature testifying to the health problems that arise from a failure in caring, whether this caring is provided informally by families or formally by paid carers.

The chapter argues that the overriding concern to maintain the public/private divide in caring work has set up a number of increasingly unsustainable paradoxes. First, there is a denial of the importance of knowledge and skill in achieving caring, despite evidence to the contrary. Second comes a recognition that care work in the family constitutes the single biggest health care institution in the country, yet there is a reluctance to study this work or to identify ways of supporting it. Third, the chapter provides a recognition of the value of this work for promoting and maintaining health, yet a complete failure to reward it. Consequently, the voices of family carers and professional carers are marginalised in social policy debates, in which their work is similarly viewed as unobtrusive and devoid of political content.

Chapter 5 considers the ways in which nurses accomplish caring in practice. It reviews the evolving literature on skills and knowledge in caring work and analyses the impact of this knowledge on the resolution of caring problems. A number of examples are given to illustrate how competencies in caring work inform practice and promote health. It demonstrates how nursing works to provide physical, tending and intimate care at the boundaries between formal and informal care, providing a practice that creates a knowledge concerning the provision of intimate care around this boundary. The chapter demonstrates how, in accomplishing this work, nurses, working in advanced health care institutions, also integrate care at the boundaries between technology and intimacy. The chapter argues that knowledge derived from working autonomously at the boundary between formal and informal care is vital both to the efficiency of modern health care institutions and to advancing health care ethically into the complex moral arena of family care. It also considers the social organisation of nursing work and identifies how the key features of caring create alternative organisational forms and structures, which are, arguably, more conducive to accomplishing caring work than are the more traditional bureaucratic and professional structures within which nursing is usually expected to operate.

Chapter 6 locates the evolution of nursing work and nursing knowledge in the multiprofessional, multi-agency arena. It reviews the current trend for organisations to be accountable to populations for the delivery of effective, integrated services rather than the delivery of a single isolated service. It acknowledges that, in taking this agenda forward, health and social care planners have recognised the overriding need to work across organisational boundaries in order to achieve effective service provision. However, in advancing this position, health and social care planners are still maintaining the, by now entrenched, traditional boundary between formal and informal care. The radicalism that informed the setting up of health and welfare services following the Second World War continues intact, leading to a perpetual reconfiguration and restructuring of services that continue to skirt the central divide between family and formal care. Again, illustrative examples are used to identify the nature of the problems facing health and social services. Examples of services that are attempting to work across the boundary of formal and informal care are reviewed and the salient features of these services identified.

Chapter 7 addresses the question of cost-effectiveness in nursing care. It reviews the substantial literature that seeks to identify the number of nurses required to provide an effective nursing service. It highlights tautologies in methodologies used to undertake research into nurse workforce planning and argues that this literature perpetuates a definition of nursing work as both unskilled and unobtrusive. The methodologies have, therefore, not kept pace with advances in nursing theory and knowledge; consequently, they perpetuate an understanding of nursing workforce requirements based on the provision of unskilled nursing designed to provide a custodial service. Nurses are thus rarely resourced enough to illustrate their potential impact on health.

Chapter 8 addresses issues of accountability and skill mix in health care. It contrasts two possible scenarios for managing the escalating demand for health care. The first scenario seeks to identify ways of reducing patient access to health care by increasing the barriers to high-technology medicine and reducing cost by upskilling health workers in order to substitute more highly paid health care workers with lower-paid workers. This is the approach adopted by most affluent industrialised societies. The second scenario recognises the proactivity of patients and their carers in determining demand for health care. It seeks to work with families in order to enable them to gain control over their health, reduce their dependency on professionals, reduce their social isolation and proactively manage their health in partnership with health and social care professionals.

In developing an analysis of accountability in nursing, Chapter 8 cautions against nursing complacency and highlights the perpetuation of 'organisational rules', nursing routines and norms of practice, which dull insight into patient problems and deny patients choice.

Chapter 9 concludes by highlighting the importance of nursing work and research at the boundary between formal and informal care. It suggests that if nurses are enabled to undertake this research, the results of this work will be central to the resolution of many of the most intransigent health and social care problems facing planners in the new millennium. In taking this agenda forward, health care providers, policy makers and planners must, however, recognise the inappropriateness of current assumptions about professionalisation and bureaucratic and hierarchical forms of control with respect to the implementation of effective caring practices. A failure to recognise the integrity of caring will lead to a failure to care and a failure to respond effectively to the total health needs of people as we enter this new century. Moreover, by not providing an environment conducive to caring, planners will fail to meet their own policy objectives to promote health while simultaneously maintaining costs. At the same time, they will remain ignorant of the causes of this policy failure.

The themes of universal and selective definitions of health introduced in the first chapter form a theoretical foundation for the book and are continued throughout each of the chapters, acting as a thread linking the different themes of the book together.

Chapter 2

Theories of Health

> The role of the health sector must move increasingly in a health promotion direction, beyond its responsibility for providing clinical and curative services. Health services need to embrace an expanded mandate which is sensitive and respects cultural needs. This mandate should support the needs of individuals and communities for a healthier life, and open channels between the health sector and broader social, political, economic and physical environmental components. (WHO, 1986)

The above quotation illustrates a fundamental shift in thinking about health care provision that forms the basis of health care policy as advocated by the World Health Organization (WHO, 1978) and the Council of Europe (1986) and, increasingly, in national European government policies (DoH, 1996a; Borst-Eilers, 1997), including that of the UK. The quote directs the health sector and those working within this sector 'to move in the direction of health promotion, beyond the provision of clinical and curative services'. Why should the health sector do this, and in particular, why and how should health care professionals fulfil this mandate? These questions are addressed in this and the next chapter. Before tackling these questions, it is, however, useful first to consider what is meant by the term 'health' so that the role of clinical and curative services in sustaining and maintaining health can be evaluated. This chapter provides an overview of contemporary definitions of health.

Health has been defined in a variety of ways; some of the definitions derive from philosophy, some from practice and some from the experience of ill-health or disability. This chapter reviews prominent definitions of health found in the literature and classifies each definition into one of two frameworks or approaches to health care provision. Definitions will be classified as either:

1. selective definitions of health that apply only to individuals who exhibit manifestations of ill-health that lead them or their family/carers to seek health care interventions;

2. universal definitions of health that apply to whole populations regardless of individual differences or manifestations of disease processes.

Selective definitions of health

Selective definitions of health tend to be derived from biomedical frameworks of health and illness and split the population into two camps:

1. those who are not currently exhibiting manifestations of illness or disease processes and are, therefore, by definition, healthy:

2. those who are exhibiting symptoms of illness and disease processes and who consequently come forward or are bought forward for health care intervention in order to restore health or ameliorate symptoms.

Three definitions of health will be classified as selective. These are described below.

Health as the absence of disease

By far the most common understanding of health is health as the absence of disease. Here, health and illness are viewed as opposite states: a person is either healthy or ill. Blaxter (1995) has shown how this definition is used extensively by the general population when they are asked how to define health. She has also demonstrated how people from all walks of life use this definition. In fact, Blaxter found people with a better education and those with a higher income used it more frequently. It was less likely to be used by those who were actually experiencing poor health or who were suffering from some long-term disability.

This dichotomous view of health is one that is extensively used by health professionals and social scientists (Seedhouse, 1986). It is useful in that it demarcates the area for professional intervention. Professional intervention is legitimised by the presence of symptoms of disease. Moreover, it is the symptoms arising from disease processes that prompt individuals or their families/carers to seek medical intervention. There is, therefore, a tacit agreement or informal contract between the patient/carer and the health care professional that a disease process has been identified and the patient/carer has agreed to the professional intervention either in order to cure or alleviate the symptoms of the disease or to manage the behaviour arising from the disease or illness.

The metaphor poignantly described by Susan Sontag (1978) is frequently used in relation to this definition of health. Here, she suggests, people are divided into two islands: those who live on the island of the healthy, who need not concern themselves with issues of health until, or only if, disease processes set in, and those who inhabit the island of the ill, whose daily lifestyles and life opportunities are circumscribed by the disease process. The illness may be a short acute episode, resulting in a short visit to the island of the sick, rather like a tourist, requiring nothing more than self-medication from the chemist and self-certificated sick leave from daily activities. Alternatively, it may be a chronic, enduring or recurrent condition requiring extensive or intensive treatment and a reconfiguring of daily activities, including work-related activities, in order to accommodate the disease process. Here, the individual is living permanently or semi-permanently on the island of the sick and, in the Sontag metaphor, forms part of the indigenous population of the island of the sick.

While neat from the point of view of defining populations and legitimising health care interventions, this dichotomy between being well and being ill does introduce a number of problems, particularly for those who are suffering from long-term or chronic disabilities, which, as the next chapter demonstrates, constitute the most prevalent forms of morbidity found in Western society.

The most important problem this raises is the spectre of social exclusion. If people have long-term or enduring conditions, they are, using this definition of health, permanently assigned to the island of the sick. Being assigned to this island has consequences for work opportunities, opportunities to acquire adequate insurance for health and pensions, and opportunities to take part in a range of social activities such as shopping and travel. As Spaink (1997), a Dutch writer who herself suffers from a chronic illness, recognises, the social constraints placed on people who are diagnosed as ill make it difficult for them to distinguish between the physical limitations imposed by the disease and the social limitations imposed by being categorised as a sufferer from a given disease. In other words, they cannot find out what they are really capable of or what their full human potential is, as they are, socially and environmentally, denied the necessary opportunities.

Perhaps more important than all of these, however, is the notion of self-stigmatisation experienced by people assigned to the island of the sick. Again, Spaink describes the self-disgust and loathing that people who have been newly diagnosed as suffering from a chronic illness can sometimes feel when presented with the diagnosis. They have to confront their own life-long prejudices against sickness associated with having always inhabited the island of the healthy. It can take some years before people realise that they have to engage in a private struggle with their own stereotypes and learn how to live comfortably and respectfully with an indigenous population with whom they had no wish to be associated.

Finally, a major problem with the definition of health as the absence of disease is that it precludes people suffering from chronic illnesses from ever being healthy. Once diagnosed, they are permanently defined as ill until such time as a cure can be realised and they can be returned to the island of the healthy. This definition has not been found to accord with the definitions of health used by people who are suffering from a chronic illness. Here, people are more likely to describe themselves as healthy apart from the disease (Blaxter, 1995) and to see health as a relative phenomenon relating to their ability to overcome or cope effectively with the disease process. People who already suffer from chronic illnesses redefine health in ways that again make it achievable.

The definition of health as the absence of disease is probably most widely used by the medical profession, who concentrate on identifying and classifying the physiological causes of disease processes in order to identify treatments that will either cure or reduce the symptoms of the disease. In so doing, medicine implies that residence on the island of the sick is temporary and that a return ticket to the island of the healthy can be acquired through the judicious use of medical technology. This definition is closely associated with biomedical interpretations of health that, according to Seedhouse (1986), portray health as a commodity that can be purchased. In other words, technology can be used to compensate for the breakdown of physiological functioning. Heart transplants, renal dialysis, surgery and drugs are all used to compensate for physiological failure. Those who have sufficient funds (either publicly or privately) can use these funds to ameliorate the inevitable physical consequences of the disease process. Cryogenics, or the freezing of bodies until a cure has been discovered or the ageing process curtailed, is probably an extreme manifestation of this definition of health.

Health as a functional capacity

In this approach, health is viewed as the capacity to fulfil essential life functions. These can include physiological functions associated with activities of daily living, such as mobility, digestion, hydration, sleep, elimination and circulation. Psychological functions include behaviour, communication and emotional stability. Social functions relate to nurturing and sustaining family members, and developing and maintaining social networks and employment (Arnold and Breen, 1998).

Health as functional capacity closely resembles Talcott Parsons' (1979) definition of health as the capacity of an individual to fulfil his or her social roles (that is, father, husband, employee, friend and so on). According to Parsons, the onset of a disease or disability reduces people's functional capacity and consequently gives rise to the need for them to adopt the 'sick role.' By adopting this role, the individual can be excused from participating in his or her normal social duties. People's absence from their social roles is tolerated so long as individuals are seen to be striving towards regaining health, which includes following medical advice.

Health as functional capacity was recognised by respondents in Blaxter's survey of lay definitions of health (Blaxter, 1995), but here the emphasis was on physiological rather than psychological or social functions. The definition was used more by elderly people, for whom the ability to perform activities of daily living was starting to become a problem and was causing them to reconsider their previously held views on health.

Arnold and Breen (1998) link concepts of adaptation to the definition of health as functional capacity, suggesting that if physical and psychological capacity are limited or diminish, the individual, family and community may have to adapt to accommodate diminished functioning. These authors point out, however, that it is often advantageous to adapt the environment to maximise functional ability. The definition of health as functional ability is also integral to concepts of rehabilitation. Here, the emphasis is on recovering the remaining capacity and maintaining maximum functioning even if that function is modified.

The definition of health as functional capacity is widely used by physiotherapists, occupational therapists, speech and language therapists and nurses in relation to individuals whose ability to undertake physical activities of daily living is temporarily or permanently impaired. Clinical psychologists and nurses, along with a range of other therapists, including art therapists, occupational therapists and speech and language therapists, may also be concerned to restore interpersonal, family and social functioning in individuals whose psychological functioning is considered to be problematic or ineffective.

Health as psychosocial adaptation or adjustment to circumstances

Psychosocial adaptation or adjustment to circumstances defines health as the ability to live a functional, happy and self-determined life within the context of one's life circumstances. It is usually used as an indicator of health rather than being a definition of health, but it is included here as it is increasingly being incorporated into a range of proxy measures for health and gives rise to a particular interpretation of appropriate health care interventions.

Psychosocial adjustment to circumstances differs from the other two selective definitions of health described above in that selectivity is not based on a disease classification, but it is selective in terms of identifying those who are having difficulty adapting and for whom interventions are necessary. In other words, a person does not have to manifest symptoms of disease processes, or inhabit the island of the sick, before this concept can be applied. People can have equal difficulty adapting to successful circumstances, such as winning the lottery, as to deprived circumstances. However, it is still based on the concept of individuals and/or families coming forward or being referred for help because they are experiencing difficulties coping with their circumstances, and intervenes only with those individuals/families who demonstrate this difficulty and for whom effective therapeutic interventions can be identified.

The importance of psychosocial adaptation to health lies in the fact that it pervades a wide range of other definitions of health, in particular the two selective definitions of health given above. Using indicators of psychosocial adaptation as an outcome measure, both of the above definitions might consider those who have successfully adapted to their circumstances, no matter how deprived, as being healthy and not in need of any further interventions, providing their basic physiological needs are being met. Consequently, therapeutic interventions are used as a means of realising health not by challenging the distribution of resources and power in society, but by providing services that will enable people living in difficult circumstances to adapt successfully to the *status quo*. Here, the concept of adjustment operates as a form of social control (Bowling, 1997).

Nursing theories of adaptation, clinical psychology and much of the work surrounding counselling and other psychodynamic therapies, such as art therapy, can be seen to incorporate the concept of psychosocial adjustment to circumstances as a basic tenet of their practice. It is, however, recognised that, for many of these health professionals, such adaptation is considered necessary if the person/family are to develop the sense of agency necessary to act autonomously to change their circumstances. This is, however, a grey area in relation to developing indicators of health. Therapeutic interventions to promote psychosocial adjustment should perhaps be viewed as one possible intervention towards achieving health, rather than as an outcome measure, which could imply that psychosocial adjustment to deprived circumstances constitutes health.

Universal definitions of health

Universal definitions of health are definitions that apply to the whole population regardless of individual differences. They tend to recognise health as a relative rather than absolute state, in which individuals strive constantly to maintain their health rather than merely being healthy. Health is, therefore, a lifelong pursuit and one that people with serious diagnostic conditions, such as ischaemic heart disease, or those who are terminally ill can still strive to achieve.

Health as growth

The concept of health as growth has it origins in developmental philosophies such as those described by Maslow (1987). Health is defined in the context of individual human endeavour. Individuals are recognised to be constantly striving towards greater knowledge, insight and understanding, culminating in Maslow's notion of self-actualisation. At this stage, people feel themselves to be autonomous, free-thinking individuals who are able to realise their own goals while maintaining a constructive relationship with their natural, cultural and familial environment. Self-actualisation is seen to be exceptional rather than common, providing a direction for development rather than a realisable goal. Maslow recognises that the achievement of higher levels of enlightenment is based on the provision of basic human necessities such as food, shelter, warmth, security and education.

Arnold and Breen (1998) have described how, within the health as growth perspective, individuals are seen as having a capacity for growth that can be nurtured and supported throughout the person's lifespan. Growth is viewed as a progressive lifelong activity, a 'striving towards' rather than a realisation of an endpoint.

Using this definition of health as growth, it is possible that those assigned to Sontag's island of the sick could realise a higher level of psychological growth, accommodation and self-actualisation than those who have not succumbed to a diagnosable physical or psychological illness. This definition of health thus integrates both populations: those who suffer from disease processes and those who do not. To this extent, therefore, it overcomes some of the problems arising from the definition of health as the absence of disease, as described above.

The close associations between health as growth and models of development can, however, create problems in the application of this definition. Arnold and Breen (1998) highlight how attempts to measure growth are frequently categorised according to life stage. Established norms are derived for each life stage (for example infancy, childhood, adolescence, early adulthood, the middle years and older years), and progress against these norms is measured. This may narrow the recognition of growth to the achievement of culturally defined personal skills at each life stage, rather than recognising the diversity in development associated with theoretical definitions of growth.

The definition of health as growth is also found to underpin some approaches to complementary therapy (Lerner, 1992), health promotion (Milz, 1992) and self-help groups (Branckaerts and Richardson, 1992).

Interestingly, health as growth was not a category identified by Blaxter in her analysis of a qualitative survey of definitions of health undertaken with the general population (Blaxter, 1995). This may be an important observation, particularly in the context of contemporary concerns with consumer views. Health as growth implies that the recipient of health care undergoes a process of change involving cognitive and/or behavioural development towards a more advanced understanding of his or her situation. This requires the health worker to use skills to facilitate growth without necessarily being able to identify what would constitute growth for that particular individual and without recourse to the limitations of socially or culturally defined norms. For people who would define themselves as healthy, using the absence of disease as the criterion for health (as the majority did in Blaxter's survey), the definition of health as growth may seem intrusive and interfering in what is essentially a private and independent progression through life.

Finally, there is very little knowledge that can be used to inform health care professionals with regard to how to facilitate growth in individual clients or population groups, other than via the selective process of working with those actively seeking psychotherapeutic health care interventions. A number of nursing theories and models seek to promote growth in relation to working with individual patients (Aggleton and Chalmers, 1986; McKenna, 1997), regardless of the underlying diagnosis or whether this type of intervention is sought by the patient. Again, these models tend to be individualised and conceptualised within a selective framework of health care provision accessed as a result of disease processes.

Health visitors, school nurses and occupational health nurses are the professional groups that come closest to using the developmental models associated with definitions of health as growth as a basis for practice. Such models are closely associated with community health clinics and welfare policies that are accessed by the whole population without any eligibility criteria being applied. The concept of universality is possibly the key concept that distinguishes the work of these health care professionals from other forms of professional health practice that tend to have their roots in selective definitions of health (Twinn and Cowley, 1992).

Health as independence, the exercise of autonomy and self-determination

Closely allied to definitions of health as growth are the concepts of health as independence, the exercise of autonomy (Doyal and Gough, 1991) and self-determination (Seedhouse, 1986). This collection of theories of health derives from humanistic traditions, which recognise that humanity is distinguished by a respect for individual self-determination and the exercise of free-will (Doyal and Gough, 1991). Seedhouse (1986), in his description of humanistic philosophies of health, discusses the concept of self-determination rather than self-actualisation. Humanistic philosophies are, he suggests, based on the principle of free choice. Without the opportunity to exercise free choice, there can be no possibility of morality. Using this collection of theories, health is a personal goal that people choose and can be different for different people. No one standard definition can be derived or applied, and multiple interpretations and choices need to be accommodated.

Like the definition of health as growth, definitions of health as the exercise of autonomy and self-determination are universal models that apply to everyone regardless of their physical or psychological state (Doyal and Gough, 1991). However, because of the predominance of selective definitions, access to social and economic resources (such as employment, educational opportunities, transport and leisure pursuits), required to underpin self-determination and the exercise of autonomy, may be denied to those who suffer from a diagnosable condition or who experience poverty, discrimination or oppression. Consequently their opportunities for realising their health may be greatly reduced within the definition of health as self-determination and the exercise of autonomy.

There are clearly close theoretical links between developmental theories of health as growth and humanistic theories of health as the exercise of autonomy or self-determination. Developmental theories are, however, explicitly based on a premise of progression towards a 'higher' level of understanding or self-actualisation, facilitated by the professional service providers, so plot a moral course or direction for health that is usually absent from theories of autonomy. Accounts of autonomy are usually framed within a context of control and rational choice, which constrain the exercise of free will and distinguish it from merely doing as one wills (Farsides, 1994). As Farsides points out, in the original Greek, *autos* means self and *nomos* means the rule of law. This recognises that for people to be described as autonomous, they need to exercise free will within a prescribed set of boundaries. Capricious or arbitrary behaviour, particularly that which damages others, is mediated by the rules within which autonomy is granted.

At a philosophical level, theories of autonomy, based on the principle of the exercise of free will within an agreed set of rules, do not necessarily imply growth or health. Instead, at an individual level, autonomy or the exercise of free will can be dogmatic, coercive, manipulative and aggressive. Because the rules and regulations governing the exercise of autonomy are frequently normative (that is, arising from social convention), autonomy can sometimes be used to justify unhealthy behaviours such as speeding on a motorway, bullying, smoking, overeating, sexism and racism. At a collective level, the concept of individual autonomy can be used to protect civil liberties against dictatorial governments and bureaucracies, as in the case of the American Constitution. The same concept can, however, also be used to justify acts of aggression such as the conquering of neighbouring territory or human rights abuses. The legal and moral debate concerning the attempted extradition from the UK to Spain of President Pinochet of Chile, to stand trial for human rights abuses, illustrates this point. The concepts of independence, autonomy and self-determination as a definition of health do not always give rise to the promotion of healthy behaviours.

Having said this, most theorists who use autonomy as a definition of health do so within a framework that allies the exercise of autonomy to concepts of morality. Seedhouse, for example, suggests that:

> A very important part of the humanist view is that self-development must be moral. It must be moral in the very broad and general sense that if a person does not wish the consequences that his self-development has for other people to happen to him, then he must not develop himself in that way. (Seedhouse, 1986, p. 52)

Similarly, Doyal and Gough (1991) locate their discussion of autonomy within a broader discussion of theories of human need. They suggest that autonomous actions that damage others cannot form the foundation of a universal theory of human need. They further point to empirical evidence that links a strong sense of self or agency and the ability to act in the world to high levels of self-esteem and altruism, suggesting that those who feel most autonomous (and therefore, using this definition, healthy) are also those most likely to act morally. This is a subjective definition of autonomy that takes little account of the objective distribution of power and the greater freedom to act (autonomy) legitimised through power structures, regardless of whether the power holder would be classified as healthy in his or her subjective feelings of autonomy, self-agency or altruism.

In using concepts such as autonomy, self-determination and independence to define health, it may be necessary to distinguish between objective and subjective definitions of autonomy. People who possess the power to exercise considerable autonomy in a social structure may not necessarily possess the personal characteristics associated with a moral use of autonomy, such as a high level of self-esteem, a subjective sense of self/agency and the ability to act in the world. Humanistic definitions of health, as autonomy exercised within a moral framework, imply that the behaviour of individuals and groups who abuse objective power or who exercise autonomy in a way that damages others within social systems could be classified as manifestations of ill-health. Sex offenders frequently fall into this category, but it could in theory be extended to include bullying and even the perpetuation of national or institutional discrimination and oppression.

Definitions of health as independence, autonomy and self-determination are found explicitly in a wide range of nursing theories.

In nursing practice, however, independence can sometimes be interpreted simply as physical or functional independence, rather than more broadly as psychological and/or social independence. A number of nursing models and theories have attempted to identify nursing interventions designed to promote independence, self-determination, autonomy and a sense of agency in situations such as palliative care or the care of people with enduring mental illness or learning disabilities. However, because of the current structure of health care provision on the basis of selectivity, nursing, except perhaps in health visiting, has rarely been able to apply these concepts universally.

Most other health care professionals would probably claim to promote independence and autonomy as a direct result of their professional intervention. Frequently, however, the definition of independence is implicit rather than explicit and functional rather than moral. In other words, the professional seeks to promote independence through the restoration of functional capacity. Interfering in how, and in the way in which, the person chooses to use the functional capacity once it has been restored would be considered to be an infringement of civil liberties and outside the remit of professional practice.

Universal definitions of health as independence, autonomy and self-determination exercised within a moral framework are difficult to operationalise within our current health care structures and culture. Consequently, our health care systems tend to focus on treating the consequences of abuses of autonomy, be this child sexual abuse or self-abuse in the form of alcoholism or drug abuse. If attempts are made to address the causes of unhealthy behaviours, the intervention usually focuses on the individual in the form of adjustment to circumstances, and occasionally on family dynamics in the form of family therapy; rarely does it engage with possible social or collective causes of these behaviours such as stigmatisation, isolation or a lack of social or personal opportunities.

In practice, health promotion officers probably come closest to struggling with this philosophical tension in their everyday practice. As Seedhouse (1997) points out, determining the ends of health promotion activities such as no smoking policies can become an abuse of civil liberties while simultaneously failing to address the causes of unhealthy behaviours such as why people smoke. Theories of autonomy and self-determination may help to promote healthy behaviour at an individual level but need to be applied universally if they are to promote a collective morality able to address social and economic inequalities in society, which are increasingly recognised as the root causes of most ill-health in society (Townsend and Davidson, 1982; Bartley *et al.*, 1997).

Health as well-being

The concept of well-being as a definition of health became prominent following its incorporation into the 1946 definition of health produced by the WHO, which stated:

> Health is a state of complete physical, mental and social well being and not merely the absence of disease and infirmity. (WHO, 1946)

This definition locates well-being as a universal construct that applies to all individuals regardless of their underlying physiological or psychological state. The concept of health as well-being gained further credibility through attempts to derive positive measures of health rather than negative measures of disease processes. A range of quality of life measures (Farquhar, 1995) has been developed in an attempt to measure well-being, and health economists have been keen to link health service costs to quality of life indicators rather than just longevity (Bowling, 1997) in order to develop alternative ways of measuring effectiveness.

Well-being is, however, an elusive term, a state that individuals experience in very different ways, making it difficult to develop a precise or objective definition. It was recognised by respondents to Blaxter's study, being defined in psychosocial terms rather than physical terms and tending to indicate a spiritual appreciation of life (Blaxter, 1995).

The link between well-being and other definitions of health that imply growth or empowerment, or even the absence of disease, is, however, difficult to establish. A temporary sense of well-being may be achieved through the use of drugs or alcohol, or through other behaviours such as domination or control, which, using alternative definitions of health (described above), may be deemed unhealthy.

Any attempt to develop well-being as a definition of health needs to relate personal experiences of well-being to healthy forms of individual and collective behaviour. Campbell (1993) has described how, for some young men, joining gangs such as skinheads and taking part in violent gang behaviour induces a sense of well-being and social cohesion that is lacking in their lives, which are otherwise characterised by social exclusion, low self-esteem and low morale. Violent behaviour would, however, rarely be advocated as an effective intervention for promoting health.

Another problem with measures of well-being is that they assume that happiness is the individual and collective goal for a given community. Philosophically, this position is difficult to justify. Human beings seek a rich tapestry of experiences during their lives and recognise that danger, grief, conflict, anger at injustice and loss form part of that experience. Some would argue that these experiences may be instrumental in promoting health as growth, as defined by Maslow (1987), or self-determination, as described by Seedhouse (1986) and discussed above. To define health exclusively as well-being denies the human need to experience loss, sorrow, grief and anger that so often accompanies people's experiences of health, illness and living.

Health economists have been the main professional group to utilise definitions of health as well-being in their work, although it is increasingly being used by a range of health care researchers to augment other outcome indicators in research.

Health as wholeness

The holistic nature of health is fundamental to concepts of healing that inform complementary medicine. Holistic approaches to health draw on many of the ideas associated with health as growth, but they do not always promote a continual striving towards self-actualisation using developmental and lifespan frameworks. Instead, holistic definitions of health tend to focus on achieving a balance between all the component parts of the system, however that system is defined. Using definitions of health derived from complementary medicine, disease or symptoms of ill health are attributed to a lack of balance in the system, and the therapist seeks to restore that balance.

As Douglas (1994) explains, although 'complementary medicine' is now the preferred term, there is a sense in which the older term of 'alternative medicine' more accurately portrayed the distinct philosophical and theoretical basis of most complementary medicine. Western medicine established its scientific basis through a process of specialisation and causal deductive analysis, which increasingly separated practice from spiritual matters. In contrast, most complementary medicine draws on ancient theories of how living beings are related to the cosmos and encompass sets of theories concerning the deep connections between psychic and physical existence (Douglas, 1994). These connections are illustrated by Hans Schaffler through a description of the ancient tradition of Ayurveda (Schaffler, 1992).

According to Schaffler, Ayurveda reveals a holistic understanding of human beings and their relationship to nature. It is seen to have an inner logic, unity and direct applicability. Ayurveda starts with the assumption that our physiology tends to compensate for homeostatic disturbances or imbalances of its own accord by creating a need for certain foods or adapting forms of behaviour. Our ability to detect this compensatory mechanism is obscured by our lifestyle, so the need frequently goes unmet, prolonging the imbalance, which ultimately damages body tissues and gives rise the onset of disease processes. Ayurveda therapists work with the patient to detect homeostatic imbalances and to correct them before the onset of irreparable physiological damage. Patients are counselled on how to restore a balance to their lifestyle and to their physiology in order to reduce imbalances thought to be the precursors of disease processes. Additional medications and nutritional supplements are occasionally prescribed in order to restore balance or ameliorate existing degenerative processes.

Ayurveda is considered to be holistic in that it embraces all human existence both in the 'vertical' plane, from concrete forms of expression through to the most abstract area of consciousness, and in the 'horizontal' plane, where it includes mind, body, behaviour and environment in its ideas and practices. According to Schaffler, Ayurveda encompasses a dynamic interpretation of health that enables practitioners to determine the effect all aspects of the internal and external environment, such as nutrition, behaviour, emotional states, climates and seasons, on an individual's psychosocial balance.

A similar claim to restore balance underpins a variety of complementary therapies (Sharma, 1994), including acupuncture, homeopathy, osteopathy, reflexology, yoga, the Alexander technique and herbalism. While some, such as osteopathy and homeopathy, focus on ameliorating existing health problems identified by the individual seeking the therapy, others, for example yoga and reflexology, would claim to have a role to play in promoting health in those who have yet to experience the onset of disease processes. Complementary medicine can, therefore, be defined as universal in its application as it can be used by individuals not experiencing any outward manifestations of disease processes, as well as individuals seeking therapeutic interventions for specific ailments.

Complementary therapy tends to focus on the individual while recognising the impact of the natural and social environment on health. An extended interpretation of health as wholeness includes an epidemiological systems analysis. This approach recognises the impact of the natural and social environment on promoting and sustaining health. The approach derives from public health and recognises the need for clean water, clean air, food and shelter as essential prerequisites to health. It incorporates an analysis of the effect of issues associated with the generation of electricity, transport policy and the distribution of wealth on individual and communal experiences of health. This approach is increasingly adopting an ecological perspective that seeks sustainable forms of energy and transportation, and the organisation of work on a human rather than global scale (Capra, 1982). The approach is manifest in the healthy cities projects (Ashton, 1992).

Holistic approaches to health have long been advocated in nursing, although nursing interpretations of holism tend to differ from those of complementary therapy and are more closely associated with systems analysis, which underpins public health. While complementary therapists focus on therapeutic diagnosis and interventions at an individual level, nursing theory has highlighted the interrelationship between physiology, psychology, social circumstances and behaviour. It has sought in its practice to compensate for an overemphasis on the physiological processes associated with biomedicine as it is practised in most Western health care settings.

Nurses have, therefore, been active in addressing issues of communication, adaptation, carer support and patient education, and in being receptive to understanding and validating the knowledge that patients and their carers gain from the daily experience of living with the illness. Nursing theory thus seeks to integrate and make sense of the multiple dimensions of the health experience as it is lived by patients and their carers. To this end, it does not always seek to instigate specific therapies, although some nurses may gain additional training in specific therapeutic techniques such as counselling or aromatherapy, or may refer patients for therapeutic interventions. The nurse–patient relationship is sometimes itself described as a form of therapy (Ersser, 1991). The lack of specific therapeutic interventions in nursing can sometimes be seen as the downfall of nursing as without such a demarcated area of expertise, it has difficulty establishing its knowledge base.

In keeping with complementary therapeutic models of holism, nursing has derived both theories of stability and balance, and theories that recognise the dynamic component of health (Leddy and Pepper, 1993). It has also incorporated concepts of growth and self-determination into its models of practice (McKee, 1991). Again, however, these theoretical models tend to focus on individuals suffering from physiological or psychological disease processes rather than using the more universal definition of growth and autonomy, described above.

Health as the realisation of potential

Health as the realisation of potential is the definition of health put forward by Seedhouse (1986). This definition, in many ways, integrates both selective and universal definitions of health. Seedhouse recognises that the full realisation of individual potential encompasses the sense of agency associated with the exercise of autonomy within a moral framework. This definition is a direction rather than an endpoint that all healthy individuals strive to achieve; hence, it includes the definition of health as growth.

For individuals suffering from disease processes, these processes present additional obstacles that have to be overcome for them to realise their potential. Those suffering from a physical illness, for example, might require additional selective medical interventions to overcome this problem, and/or functional interventions to maintain or restore functional capacity. They may, however, be more than able, if this problem is adequately addressed, to fulfil their academic potential. Conversely, people with full physical health may experience psychological obstacles to learning or motivation that are preventing them realising their academic potential. Work for health would seek a range of selective interventions to reduce these obstacles.

According to Seedhouse (1986), health is stratified by genetic endowment but should not be stratified by environmental or social conditions. Work for health is about striving to reduce the obstacles that prevent a person realising his or her full physical and psychological potential. The more physical and psychological problems people have, the more input they are going to need to overcome the obstacles to realising their potential. Interventions are selectively applied to individuals according to an identification of the particular configuration of obstacles preventing them realising their full potential.

However, while work at an individual level is of necessity selective, in working to create situations in which individuals can realise their full potential, Seedhouse suggests, work for health must address and overcome the obstacles to health embedded in social and political structures, including oppression and domination. Health as the realisation of potential, therefore, also includes a whole systems approach in working to overcome the structural obstacles embedded in social systems that prevent people realising their full potential regardless of their individual physical and psychological state.

The definition of health as the realisation of potential develops an integrated, inclusive approach to health care provision that combines selective professional expertise with more universal, collective approaches. There is still, however, a tendency to locate responsibility for health with health care providers and professionals within this approach. While the importance of the community dimension to health is acknowledged, health as the realisation of potential tends to advocate primarily an educational approach rather than a democratic, participatory approach designed to unleash the power of the community to determine its own destiny.

Health as empowerment

Health as empowerment is rooted in a recognition of the strong link between individuals' and communities' sense of power and the level of health they experience (Arnold and Breen, 1998). At one level, health as empowerment builds on developmental theories of health as growth and humanistic theories of health as self-determination and the exercise of autonomy. It recognises that work for health needs actively to transfer power to individuals and communities in order to promote a sense of control over destiny and, therefore, promote health. Theories of health as growth and health as autonomy, while applying to whole populations, tend to focus on individual growth and autonomy. Health as empowerment, however, invariably encompasses a community or collective perspective and often focuses on facilitating participation in political processes by individuals and communities normally denied access to these processes (Oakley, 1989).

The origins of health as empowerment can be traced to two sources: one is the community development models emerging from developing countries (Oakley, 1989); the other is derived from feminist perspectives on collective action (MacDonald, 1998). Health care in developing countries has had to recognise that the overwhelming majority of the world's people have no regular access to organised and professionally based health services. In coping with the problems of staying alive and combating disease, millions of people are totally dependent on their own efforts and initiative. Developing countries are increasingly recognising that it is unrealistic and hugely time-consuming to adopt policies for improving health that require the introduction of Western-style medical and health services. Instead, community participation and engagement in health policies has been seen as a more effective and rapid vehicle for improving health across large sectors of the world's poorest people (Sanders, 1985; Oakley, 1989).

Feminist writers have also contributed to the health as empowerment debate. Feminists have criticised the mystification of the processes of the health, disease and treatments associated with professional approaches to health care provision. They have sought to disseminate knowledge about physiological processes and disease processes through publications and magazines in a language that can be understood by ordinary people. They have encouraged individuals to take control of medical processes and remain in control of their own bodies.

Feminist analysis has also recognised the important role of the community in sustaining and maintaining health. Women are now generally recognised as the gatekeepers of their own health and that of their families (Graham, 1984). Family health is linked to environmental community living conditions, poor housing, a lack of safe play areas for children, heavy inner city traffic and other daily living hazards, all of which have been recognised as contributing to health problems and requiring collective political action for change to occur (Rice *et al.*, 1992).

Health as empowerment thus links community health policies in developing countries with similar movements in the developed world. Both movements are responding to recognised deficiencies in the traditional form of health care provision found in the Western health care sector. Interestingly, the rhetoric, if not the reality, of health as empowerment has seeped into government agendas, and many of the principles underpinning health as empowerment form the basis of contemporary health care policy. This is particularly the case in relation to the development of health action zones (HAZs) in the UK, which aim to improve the collective health of a total community by a combination of community participation and the promotion of health-sustaining public policies that encompass transport, housing and industry as well as the traditional health and social services (DoH, 1998a).

One possible explanation for this can be traced to the recognition that health as empowerment unties the knot of dependency that characterises much health work (Oakley, 1989). Ultimately, health care provision that promotes a passive dependency on interventions by health care professionals is increasingly expensive to sustain and, in the face of our contemporary understanding of processes for sustaining health, largely ineffective. As the Council of Europe recognises, there is 'a realisation that spectacular advances in medicine bring with them a return on investment which is disappointing, when looked at in terms of population health. They have almost always involved increasing costs for diminishing returns' (Council of Europe, 1986, p. 9).

Community empowerment, in shifting the locus of power from health professionals to local communities, has the advantage of reducing dependency on health professionals while increasing effective preventative self-care processes on the part of those communities. This approach is considered to be more sustainable than continued dependence on a professionally dominated tertiary health service. It is perhaps this principle that unites health policy in the developing world and the developed world, and underpins a range of international and national policies, including the Alma Ata, the Ottawa Charter and the Health of the Nation.

However, while the principle of the empowerment of local communities by participation may have been accepted in health, the interpretation and meaning attached to this vary widely. There are many versions of community participation in health that maintain the dominance of health professionals over the health care agenda (Oakley, 1989). At the heart of the problem lies the need to increase knowledge and public awareness of the types of behaviours and self-care management known to support health, for example immunisation, clean water and maintaining sewage disposal, while simultaneously encouraging the community to take control of this agenda for themselves. In reality, the local community might perhaps be more concerned about other issues not seen as central by health care providers or within their remit to remedy.

Social workers have perhaps been the main group of professionals to encompass concepts of community empowerment in their practice, largely because a large portion of their work is located with disadvantaged and vulnerable groups of people. Health visitors may also become involved in this type of activity. Much of this work is undertaken by non-health care professionals such as local women's groups or voluntary organisations. Patient self-help groups and advocacy groups are also involved in this area.

Summary and conclusion

This chapter has reviewed two main approaches to classifying definitions of health: a selective approach that defines health as the absence of diagnosable disease and/or the promotion of functional capacity to enable individuals to adapt successfully to their circumstances, and a universal approach that locates health as a lifelong pursuit.

Selective social policies tend to be associated with individualised approaches to public service provision that incorporate some form of rationing based on a measure of need, such as means testing. In the case of health being debated here, it is suggested that selective definitions of health ration access to health care based on evidence of demonstrable disease processes that indicate a need for health care interventions.

Increasingly, it is suggested that this access should be mediated by evidence that the intervention is cost-effective in ameliorating the symptoms or causes of the disease (Sackett and Haynes, 1995). It is recognised that once a disease process has been identified, access to care is universal – but only for those deemed to be in need in the first instance.

Conversely, the universal definitions of health being suggested here apply to the whole population regardless of each individual's underlying mental or physical capacity. Some needs assessment may be undertaken within a universal service in order to compensate for additional health care needs arising from disease processes. However, within universal definitions of health, it is recognised that no individual is exempt from the impact of health care policies and strategies designed to promote health. Neither are individuals exempt from taking responsibility not only for their own health, but also for the health of others.

The selective definition of health – as the absence of disease and, in the face of disease, the promotion of functional capacity and adjustment to circumstances – is perhaps the most prevalent definition of health found in Western health care. Unsurprisingly, this definition is also held by the majority of the population who have yet to experience a long-term illness or disability. This definition enjoys widespread support, provides a clear set of parameters for identifying the population in need of health care interventions and defines the boundaries of health care provision. It also forms the basis of a legitimate contract between the patient seeking help to ameliorate physical or psychological symptoms and the health care practitioner providing interventions.

Universal definitions of health are much more difficult to use as the basis for intervention strategies. They apply general principles to the whole population, although they can locate specific obstacles to health experienced by subsections of the population and prioritise the removal of those obstacles for this group. The basis for intervention is less clear as it is not based on a voluntary contract initiated by the patient or service user. The strategies used may seem invasive of privacy and undermining to those in receipt of services. Clear indicators of health using universal definitions have yet to be devised, so problems arise in monitoring effectiveness of service provision. Behaviours that in other circumstances may be considered successful, such as bullying and domination, are increasingly being defined as unhealthy, and this could prove to be controversial. Community participation is more and more being advocated as a process for sustaining and integrating health into the everyday lives of the general population, but no clear understanding of how this can be effectively achieved has yet emerged.

The use of selective and universal definitions of health in professional practice

From the above discussion, it is apparent that the overwhelming majority of health care professionals practise within a selective framework of health care provision. The extent to which it is possible for professional groups to implement universal health care policies is clearly constrained by the structural environment in which they work. However, in order to evaluate the contribution that different professional groups could potentially make to the promotion of selective or universal health care policies, it is not perhaps their practice that should be examined, but the theoretical models and frameworks for developing practice that should form the focus of attention.

Selective approaches to health care provision arise out of a categorisation of need for health care based on evidence of diagnosable disease. Selective health care policies, therefore, map directly onto biomedical models of provision. Models of professional practice based on a restoration or maintenance of physical and/or psychological functional capacity also imply a selective approach to health care provision. These models predominate among nurses, physiotherapists, doctors, occupational therapists, psychologists, art therapists and speech and language therapists. In fact, these models are found almost universally across all health care professionals.

Universal definitions of health tend to focus on global concepts such as growth, autonomy and the realisation of potential. It is undeniably the case that selective health care policies are an essential component of any health care system seeking to promote these ends. Many health care professionals would in fact claim that these are the ends that they are pursuing for their patients. With the exception of health visiting, school nursing and social work, most models of health care practice fail to distinguish between functional independence and the exercise of independence or autonomy within a moral framework that includes both theories of growth and self-development and theories of community empowerment.

Public health perspectives have highlighted the importance of the physical environment in sustaining the health of whole populations. The whole systems approach offered by nursing and health visiting has begun to bridge the gap between the islands of the healthy and the sick by recognising the impact that ill-health makes on those who are healthy in the form of the imperative to care (McCubbin and McCubbin, 1993;

Twigg and Atkin, 1994) and in identifying ways of reintegrating the sick back into mainstream society (Robinson and Elkan, 1997).

For example, school nursing and community children's nursing play a crucial role in facilitating normal educational processes for children with physical and mental learning difficulties. Other professional groups also working to this end include occupational therapists and play therapists, but nursing tends to be distinguished by its advocacy role within the wider social system. Nurses will and frequently do address individual classes and whole schools on the special needs of a sick child and the ways in which other pupils and teachers can help. This type of activity arguably promotes, among groups of individuals not currently experiencing disease processes, a growth in understanding of health care issues and an imperative to take responsibility for the health care needs of others. This promotes a more universal understanding of the collective nature of health and the sustaining of health in society. Through the advocacy process, the problem is not individualised but is located in a collective understanding of health care needs associated with universal definitions of health.

This chapter has reviewed current definitions of health. It has distinguished between selective and universal definitions of health and illustrated the dominance of selective definitions of health deriving from biomedical perspectives on the structure and culture of health care provision. It has provided evidence suggesting that selective definitions of health are also used extensively by members of the general public in determining their understanding of health and health care provision. Universal definitions of health, while providing a framework for health promotion, are marginalised within the current health sector and are very difficult for health professionals to implement. This is the case even in those situations such as nursing, health visiting, social work and health promotion, which explicitly use universal definitions in their theories and models of practice.

Given these difficulties, it is unsurprising that selective policies continue to dominate health care provision. There has, however, been a widespread recognition of the need to move towards more universal definitions of health in the provision of health services. The next chapter reviews some of the evidence underpinning this policy direction and addresses the question of why, and in whose interests it is, to adopt such policies.

Chapter 3

Trends in Health and Illness

'Moving beyond the provision of clinical and curative services', as suggested by contemporary European and WHO policies, must sometimes seem remote and far removed from the everyday experience of busy nurses and other health care practitioners working in increasingly pressurised hospital wards and departments – a window on somebody else's responsibility rather than theirs. For many practitioners and health care providers, the question is how to reduce demand for services by increasing rationing and selectivity, rather than how to increase demand by moving to the provision of universal services.

Are the principles of universal health care, of health promotion, the development of personal skills, the creation of health in everyday environments, home, work, leisure, and the empowerment of local communities of relevance to people working in the technically advanced health sectors of the developed world? How, if at all, does universal health care link to government policies that promote primary health care and push already overburdened health care practitioners to take on an even wider remit than the one they are currently addressing? How and why should health care practitioners address this remit? This chapter considers these questions.

Are universal definitions of health of relevance to people working in the technically advanced health sectors of the developed world?

Modern health care in the developed world is dominated by advanced technology, increasing technological innovation and a focus on hospital-based medical interventions, as is much health care in developing countries. Newsom-Davis and Weatherall (1994) have high-lighted the impact of advances in transplantation, the human genome project, cancer therapies, psychopharmacology and new vaccines, to name but a few, that are going to dominate the early part of this millennium. At the same time, millions of people across the globe continue to die from preventable diseases such as water-borne infectious diseases and malnutrition (Sanders, 1985). There is, therefore, a steep global gradient between those who have access to a range of technologies for health and those who are denied access to even basic ones. These range from individual technologies associated with medicine such as heart transplants to the communal ones that produce a clean water supply, sanitation or a nutritious diet.

Medical technology tends to be concentrated in hospitals, which, in most countries, form the focal point for diagnosis, treatment and, importantly, training health care practitioners. There is, however, very little evidence that a hospital-dominated health care system is effective in improving the overall health of the population.

In a now classical historical study, McKeown (1979) charted the impact of medical interventions on improvements in mortality and morbidity in England from the middle of the 19th century to the middle of the 20th century. He concluded that the major factors accounting for most of the decline in mortality during that period were: a decline in family size; improvements in sanitation; better nutrition brought about by lower food prices, which were the result of new technology in agriculture increasing productivity and advances improving food distribution; and improvements in the standard of living and housing. Medical interventions did not start to affect mortality rates until the introduction of antibiotics in 1945. By this time, a substantial reduction in mortality from the major killers of the 19th century, including tuberculosis, cholera, diphtheria and dysentery, had already been achieved.

Other factors found to be important in reducing mortality were female literacy (Williams, 1986), slum clearance programmes and access to sterilised milk (Atkins, 1992). Oakley (1984) has demonstrated how maternal mortality rates did not fall significantly until improvements in living standards, greater equality and food rationing were introduced during and after the Second World War.

Early epidemiological studies highlighted the importance of clean water, air and the safe disposal of sewage for improving the health of the population. In contrast, contemporary epidemiology reveals the importance of early life experiences in determining health in middle and old age (Essen and Wedge, 1982; DSS, 1988 [Acheson Report]; Blane *et al.*, 1996). Bartley *et al.* (1997) highlight how, as individuals progress through life, there are critical periods when they are at risk of acquiring attributes or experiences that predispose towards illness. Critical life course events and predisposing factors include: intergenerational factors such as maternal nutrition during pregnancy (Barker, 1992), unemployment, job insecurity, the onset of chronic illness and exit from the labour market. Without support from appropriate health and social policies, these events can have adverse effects on future patterns of individual and community health.

In reviewing the evidence, Bartley *et al.* (1997, p. 1194) conclude, 'Living conditions cannot simply be left to fluctuate as people pass through childhood and their reproductive and working years and into old age, because health and quality of life at any one stage is affected by prior circumstances and events.' Evidence such as this tends to reinforce the comment made by Archie Cochrane and his colleagues that 'health service factors are relatively unimportant in explaining the differences in mortality between developed countries' (Cochrane *et al.*, 1978, p. 205).

What has remained consistent over time, however, is the social distribution of health and illness, which in the UK has changed remarkably little despite the health and social reforms of the post-Second World War era (Charlton and Murphy, 1997). The Black Report (Townsend and Davidson, 1982) used essentially official statistics of England and Wales in the early 1970s and demonstrated 'that men and women in occupational class V had a two-and-a-half times greater chance of dying before reaching retirement age than their professional counterparts in occupational class I' (Townsend and Davidson, 1982, p. 51). The report also found that if this statistic were broken down by age, this difference was a constant feature of the entire human lifespan. Mortality was found to be higher at birth and during the first year of life, in childhood, adolescence and adult life for people in occupational class V compared with those in occupational class I. Townsend and Davidson (1982) state that 'At any age people in occupational class V have a higher rate of death than their better off counterparts' (p. 51). These differences have long been recognised.

What the Black Report demonstrated was that, despite all the health and social policy interventions that marked out the post-Second World War era in the UK, this gap was widening: 'the difference in [mortality] rate between the lowest classes (IV and V combined) and the highest (I and II combined) actually increased between 1959–63 and 1970–72' (Townsend and Davidson, 1982, p. 206). The Black Report concluded that poverty and deprivation were the principal causes of the premature death and lesser life expectancy of the lowest social classes. Similar patterns have been found in other developed countries, including the USA (Abel-Smith, 1994; Flaskerud and Winslow, 1998).

Moser *et al.* (1990) demonstrated that the average rise of real income between 1979 and 1987 in the UK was 23.1 per cent. However, the rise for the bottom 10 per cent of the population was 0.1 per cent, that for the next 10 per cent was 2.4 per cent and that for the next 10 per cent, 2.8 per cent. During this period, the proportion of children living on or below the poverty line, defined here as living on less than half the average income, rose from 12 per cent to 26 per cent. Increasing numbers of single mothers (whether unmarried, divorced or separated), elderly people, seriously disabled people and the chronically unemployed are also living on or below the poverty line. The impact of these findings for the health of the UK population is illustrated in a comparative study of income distribution and inequalities in health undertaken by Bradshaw (1994), who found that those countries which had narrowed their income distribution achieved similar reductions in inequalities in health.

Accumulated evidence of the impact of socio-economic factors on health has led Grossman (1972) to propose the model of health outlined in Figure 3.1.

Grossman's model portrays the number of healthy life years that a person can expect depending on the level of socio-economic support he or she receives throughout life across a broad range of factors. Health in its broadest sense is the product not of health services, but of access to

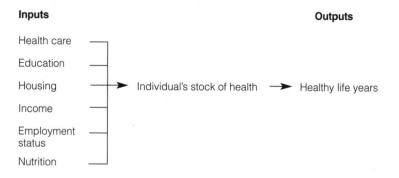

Figure 3.1   Grossman's models of factors influencing health

a broad range of social supports that cumulatively give rise to the number of healthy life years a person can expect and simultaneously reduce the need for curative intervention services.

From the evidence cited above, however, it would seem that, for busy nurses and health care practitioners working in the health sector, the combination of the widening inequality gap and advances in technology means that their daily workload looks set to continue unabated or even increase. Given this scenario, health care practitioners are going to find it difficult to do little more than increase the pace at which they work, and increase selectivity by reducing access and increasing rationing in order to keep abreast of the growing demand. Moreover, the increasing demand for health services may not come primarily from the most disadvantaged sections of society. The advent of new technologies and drugs means that, unlike the situation in the period that McKeown studied, more and more treatments are now effective at maintaining life, if not curing the underlying physiological causes of ill-health. In such circumstances, it is the relatively affluent sections of society who increase their demand for health care as they are aware of the benefits of health care in improving the quality of life.

Tackling the problems at source, linking into the community and introducing preventative strategies, while welcomed in principle by many health care practitioners, frequently has to be undertaken in a hectic working environment in which opportunities for planning and implementing new working practices are few. Moreover, the strategic shifts recommended in documents such as the Ottawa Charter (WHO, 1986), while based on sound epidemiological evidence, are often contrary to the daily demands experienced by health care practitioners. Quite how practitioners are expected to undertake a shift in their practice towards the principles outlined in the Ottawa Charter is rarely clarified.

Do universal definitions of health underpin government policies that promote primary health care?

The historical emphasis on hospitals as the focal point for health care provision reflects a number of diverse factors. Many modern-day hospitals originated from charitable foundations and religious orders, or from the custodial policies towards the poor and mentally ill pursued in earlier times. More recently, hospitals have been planned and developed as cost-effective centres for providing expensive, technically advanced care.

Abel-Smith (1994) points to the large number of highly trained staff, including technical and managerial staff as well as health professionals, required in modern-day health care to ensure that patients receive the right technological interventions at the right time in a safe and informed environment. The complexity associated with much modern-day health technologies means that access to the necessary expertise to support investigations and medical interventions can be more easily managed within a hospital environment. Hospitals provide economies of scale and improve efficiency by bringing the patients to the techno-logical centre rather than taking the technology out to the population. Safety and standards of care can be more easily monitored within a hospital environment. Given the increasing advances in medical tech-nology highlighted by Newsom-Davis and Weatherall (1994), the demand for hospitals and the efficiencies associated with hospitals are unlikely to diminish.

However, identifying exactly how many hospital beds to provide and where these should be located remain important and frequently unresolved problems. It is now widely recognised that the principle first observed by Roemer, that the supply of hospital beds largely determines demand, holds true in most situations. 'The more hospital beds are provided the more they will be used. Roemer's law' (Abel-Smith, 1994, p. 136).

Clarke (1996), in a review of the length of hospital stay literature, found that reductions in length of stay only reduce hospital costs if wards or hospitals are simultaneously closed. Without the direct with-drawal of services in this way, reducing length of stay while maximising bed occupancy simply increases hospital throughput. In other words, either more patients are treated for a shorter period of time or the same patients are recycled more frequently through hospital facilities. In practice, reducing length of stay while main-taining bed supply and a high bed occupancy will probably do both. It is likely to increase access for patients previously denied access while simultaneously increasing the readmission rate. It is not, however, likely to reduce cost as most of the costs associated with admission to hospital occur in the immediate post-admission period (when most of the investigations are conducted and referrals made) and gradually reduce the longer the patient is in hospital. In these circumstances, a reduction in length of stay, which increases the number of readmis-sions or new patients seen, is likely to increase hospital costs if both bed supply and occupancy remain unchanged.

Clarke (1996) found that, in surgical wards, a reduction in length of stay following surgery, without a reduction in bed supply, led to an increase in the number of patients on whom surgery was performed. She pointed out that either patients were going untreated prior to the reduction in length of stay, or unnecessary surgical operations were being performed following the reduction in length of stay in order to keep the bed occupancy up. She concluded that 'The benefits of a person's reduced time in hospital are critically dependent on the effectiveness and appropriateness of the work which fills up the slack' (Clarke, 1996, p. 177).

Most of the literature on discharging patients from hospital assumes that the consultant is the key decision maker. Indeed, many of the reductions in length of stay have been introduced following audits that have revealed widely differing lengths of stay for patients receiving similar treatments and having a similar type of illness. Despite this convention, however, Clarke (1996) found strong evidence from two studies to suggest that individual consultants do not determine length of stay. She states that 'Surprisingly, it has been suggested that there is a "when in Rome do what the Romans do" effect on consultants which determines their patients' length of stay in any given hospital' (Clarke, 1996, p. 174).

This illustrates how, despite assuming power to determine discharge processes and in particular length of stay, consultants' decision making may be constrained by the availability and organisation of other health care professional and social service inputs. The local configuration of health and social care, especially the availability of beds, may be more important in determining length of stay and creating the 'culture of Rome' within which consultants have to operate than are the purely medical decisions assumed to determine access to hospital resources.

So what is accounting for the increasing costs of health care identified across the world? Donaldson and Gerard (1993) point to the link between gross domestic product and health care spending. In most countries access to health services depends on the identification of a disease process. Once such a process is identified each nation spends what it can afford. Increases in health care spending correspond to increases in economic growth. Abel-Smith (1994) suggests that the ageing of the population has been too small to date to account for more than a small part of the rising cost of health care. He identifies the increasing cost of new technology as the common feature throughout the world in explaining the increasing costs of health care globally. It follows that determining the supply of new technology is fundamental to ensuring that it is used appropriately and efficiently. As with hospital beds, the more technology that is available, the more it will be used without any necessary correlation to improvements in health outcomes. Too reduced a supply of technology is, however, likely to curtail access to the more privileged sections of society and to deny access to the more vulnerable sections of the population who consistently demonstrate the greatest levels of ill-health. This pattern has been repeatedly demonstrated in both developed and developing countries (Sanders, 1985; Abel-Smith, 1994).

Abel-Smith goes on to suggest that, in developed countries, the key problems facing health care providers are unnecessary admission to hospital, excessive length of stay, the excessive use of diagnostic tests, irrational prescribing and overprescribing. The same problems are found in some developing countries. He suggests that reducing hospital costs depends on maximising the number of day surgery cases, providing adequate cheaper alternatives in either other institutions, for example residential/nursing homes for elderly, or patients' own homes. The separate financing of alternative forms of provision from different and often less glamorous budgets creates barriers to the implementation of policies designed to reduce the excessive and ineffective use of hospital beds.

None of the problems identified by Abel-Smith as being paramount in developed countries seems to reflect the principles underpinning universal definitions of health described in the previous chapter. Instead, the issues highlighted by Abel-Smith concern efficiency, defined as treating people with a level of skill and resource appropriate to their need, that is, for example, not keeping elderly people in hospital for want of a residential or nursing home place; not keeping people in hospital awaiting the outcome of diagnostic tests; and not using skilled nurses to deliver food to ambulant and orientated hospital patients who simply require hotel-type services.

Primary care in the UK is usually associated with the generalist services provided by a general medical practitioner or GP. Abel-Smith describes primary care hospitals as hospitals staffed by doctors without specialist qualifications. It is important, therefore, to distinguish between primary care and welfare or community care. Primary care tends to refer to the provision of some form of medical service based on evidence of symptoms of ill-health, whereas welfare implies a more universal bottom-up approach to health encompassing the whole community and ensuring access to knowledge on health promotion and disease prevention. The infant welfare clinics provided by local authorities from 1918 onwards in the UK are an example of the latter.

The distinction between primary care and community care is an important one that frequently gets lost in the rhetoric surrounding contemporary health care policies. In discussing the current emphasis on primary care, Abel-Smith highlights five underlying factors:

1. The importance of intersectoral action for health development and the evidence of a widening health and income gap that confounded economic predictions of improvements in health arising from overall improvements in national and individual prosperity.

2. The recognition by the WHO that combatting infectious diseases was more effectively achieved through general improvements in sanitation, environmental health, education, nutrition and clean water than through single-disease campaigns. Similar claims can be made for combatting the major diseases of the developed world. Here, it is now recognised that reducing obesity, increasing exercise and improving diet helps to prevent the onset of major killers such as heart disease, stroke and hypertension, as well as reducing the incidence of enduring illnesses such as diabetes (Charlton and Murray, 1997).

3. Health care practice and the financing of health care tend to divide preventative and promotive health care from curative action. This reflects the historical division between prevention and promotion as a collective activity, and curative action as an individual activity. This division means that health care professionals do not necessarily need to concern themselves with prevention and health promotion, while the health care industry focuses almost exclusively on the provision of curative services. This division is formalised under systems of health insurance, which seek to define exactly what is and is not covered in the policy. Such a situation will be familiar to most health care practitioners and presents one of the major obstacles to adopting practices that incorporate prevention and health promotion as central aspects of professional practice.

4. There is increasing evidence of a range of relatively cheap and effective health care activities that do not reach millions of people throughout the world. Instead, increasing amounts of health care resources are concentrated on the relatively privileged minorities in both developing and developed countries. The utilisation of these resources by privileged minorities makes little impact on improving the overall health of the population.

5. Finally, there is a concern that health care professionals have appropriated health from the people and mystified the process by which it can be achieved and sustained. This is based on the assumption that health is a social commodity rather than a commodity that can be monopolised by professionals and then rationed for their personal profit.

Collectively, these factors make the case not just for a shift to a primary care-led NHS, but also for the development of community-based welfare policies designed to give the control of health back to local communities, as described in the universal definitions of health given in the previous chapter. There is, however, some evidence that the shift to primary care in the UK is also about attempting to control the escalating costs of hospital-based health care by introducing a knowledgeable purchaser to act on behalf of the consumer in purchasing hospital services and ensuring standards of provision. There is very little in the purchasing arrangements that would challenge the current distribution of health care resources; indeed, it may even reduce access for chronically ill or vulnerable sections of the population who may appear to be too expensive to be included in fund-holders' purchasing agreements. Whether this proves to be the case under purchasing arrangements arising from primary care groups remains to be seen.

The shift to primary care entailed in much recent government legislation seems conservative and designed to reduce costs and contain workload rather than introduce any radical change in the ideologies underpinning health care provision. It is possible to suggest that moves to primary care, enshrined in much government legislation in the UK, are designed to put checks and balances into the system and to introduce incentives for using existing resources more efficiently. Legislation aims to increase productivity and enable health care providers to cope with extra demand without a massive rise in cost.

Why should health care practitioners address the remit arising from universal definitions of health?

The emphasis on reducing hospital costs that seems to dominate the current health care agenda may, in the short term, introduce sufficient innovations in service delivery to manage increasing demand without a similar increase in the supply of health services. However, it is questionable how far this can be sustained, particularly in the light of escalating advances in medical technology that seem always to demand the concentration of highly skilled staff in order to ensure their effective use by the privileged minority of the population.

Another approach to thinking about the management of medical technology is, perhaps, to understand the management of medical technology and health service provision in the context of contemporary patterns of disease in developed countries.

There is evidence that, although social class differences remain, the health and welfare reforms of the 20th century in developed countries have been successful in improving the overall health of the population. Expectation of life at birth is a hypothetical measure that describes the average number of years a newborn baby can be expected to live if the current mortality rate continues to apply. It is aggregated across the whole population so, for example, an increase in infant mortality will have a marked effect on reducing life expectancy, as will an increase in premature mortality in any one section of the total population. It, therefore, provides an indicator of the direction of health trends over time. In the UK, expectation of life at birth has risen from 44 years for men and 47 years for women around the turn of the century to 73 and 78 years respectively in 1988–1990 (Walford, 1994). Life expectancy is continuing to rise and, with the exception of young males, for whom mortality rates are rising, it is not clear when it will level off (Charlton, 1997; DoH, 1997).

While people might be living longer, this increase in life expectancy has not been matched by an increase in disability-free life expectancy. In other words, although people are living longer, they are also more sick for an increasing length of time (Bebbington, 1991). Grundy (1997) debates the reasons for this. It is unclear whether future improvements in health using universal policies will not improve life expectancy, but will compress experience of chronic ill-health to a very short timespan, just preceding death, or whether life expectancy will continue to rise but will be unevenly distributed across the population, with an increase in inequalities in life expectancy for different sections of the population (Fries, 1980). Grundy concurs with Manton (1982), who suggests that there is a dynamic relationship between mortality and morbidity bought about by medical interventions that slow the rate of degeneration in chronic illness and thus prolong life.

Charlton *et al.* (1997) point to evidence from the USA suggesting that clinical preventative and curative services have contributed about five years to the increase in life expectancy this century, when averaged over the whole population, and have the potential to add another two years if therapies already known to be effective are extended to more people.

Grundy (1997) also highlights evidence of a reduction in the extent of serious disability and a marked drop in the proportion of people unable to undertake four activities of daily living without assistance. This, she suggests, could be attributable to a change in the management of illness and an increasing recognition that bedrest is generally dangerous rather than beneficial.

There appear, therefore, to be twin pressures acting on health services. The first is managing safe, regulated and equitable access to the rapidly expanding portfolio of medical technology, the second expanding access to the range of universal social support services required to ensure an equitable distribution of health within and between populations. The Alma Ata declaration (WHO, 1978) and the Ottawa Charter (WHO, 1986) both recognise that promoting disability-free life years is dependent on nations effectively managing the second pressure, that is, ensuring access to the wide range of universally available social support services necessary to promote health, as depicted in the Grossman model (p. 34). It is only if this is achieved that it will be possible to contain and equitably distribute access to medical technology. Any failure in community health will give rise to an increasing pressure on hospitals to compensate at a tertiary level for inequalities in access to primary resources. The types of technological intervention that hospitals have the expertise to offer may not, however, be the most effective way of responding to the health care needs of the presenting population.

Globally, it has been estimated that 54 million people die each year, nearly half from a chronic health problem. Among adults, the leading causes are circulatory disease (heart disease and stroke), cancer and chronic pulmonary illness (WHO, 1997a). Morbidity and mortality from chronic degenerative diseases tends to be more prevalent in the developed world where more traditional causes of death from malnutrition and water- and air-borne infections have been reduced. There is, however, evidence that in developing countries, where people are surviving into adulthood they are acquiring the same disease patterns as are found in the developed world.

From a clinical perspective, what is striking about cardiovascular disease and respiratory disease is that they tend to be chronic and degenerative diseases. Technological developments in the treatment of cancer means that this disease is now being categorised as a chronic illness rather than a terminal illness. Mental illness does not seem to respond to either prevention or high-technology interventions, beyond the alleviation of some symptoms, but it does respond to a combination of health and social service inputs designed to improve social functioning and quality of life (Walford, 1994).

A key feature of chronic and degenerative diseases is that they are enduring. This simple phrase belies a host of complex issues facing health care professionals. Not only do chronic degenerative diseases arise from the accumulated effects of the genetic, physiological, psychological, cultural, environmental and social history of the individual concerned, but they also largely determine the future life course of the patient within this complex milieu.

In a discussion of the health care needs of people suffering from chronic illnesses, Pott (1992) has identified four major issues:

1. Chronically ill people need to know how the illness will develop and what it means for their life. This means that health care professionals need to use psychological and psychosomatic knowledge, which provides a theoretical basis for intervention.

2. The chronically ill person has to learn to accept the illness. This is a particularly difficult problem in a society that stigmatises illness, often causing sufferers to self-stigmatise (Schnurre, 1992; Spaink, 1997). The problem is not helped by a health care system that often still assumes cure to be a realisable outcome (even if it is not currently available but depends on further research) and interprets a failure to be cured as a failure on the part of the patient to, for example, comply with medical prescriptions. It is compounded by a society that makes clear demarcations between people who are deemed to be healthy and fit, who are to be included in employment, insurance and many other aspects of life, and those who are labelled ill and, by definition, denied access to a wide range of social and economic opportunities.

3. The chronically ill person needs support to cope with the restrictions, the isolation and the disruption of social contacts resulting from a chronic illness, otherwise further illnesses may develop. The provision of small networks, social support and self-help is a key requirement for the quality of life of the chronically ill person, who depends on voluntary care and personal contact. These are important areas in which an understanding of health promotion for the chronically ill is crucial.

4. Finally, there is the need for co-operation and co-ordination between the many different agencies supporting the chronically ill, including benefits agencies as well as health and social care agencies.

What is apparent from Pott's summary of the issues facing the chronically ill is that, as individuals, patients have an active role to play in sustaining a healthy life while living out their remaining years with a chronic condition. Recognising and helping patients to be proactive in the management of their illness requires health care professionals to understand the illness as the patient is experiencing it, as well as understanding the optimum medical outcome that can be achieved by expert technical intervention. Within our current health care system, this is a complex task as it would seem that achieving optimum health care outcome derives from a mixture of both a quantitative and a qualitative understanding of the patient's condition.

This can be illustrated with reference to the prevention and management of stroke. It is well established that the main risk factor for stroke is raised blood pressure (Charlton *et al.*, 1997), which can be reduced by a change in lifestyle (for example, cessation of smoking, weight reduction and better nutrition) and by the early detection and treatment of hypertension. There is considerable evidence from clinical trials that mortality from stroke can be reduced by half with intensive antihypertensive treatment. Both Walford (1994) and Charlton *et al.* (1997) cite the findings of a confidential enquiry into stroke deaths in a single health district in England. The enquiry found that there were avoidable factors in 29 per cent of the 123 deaths examined. The main avoidable factors were a failure of hypertensive patients to stop smoking and a failure of adequate follow-up and treatment of hypertension.

Addressing these factors requires health care professionals to understand the patient's experience of the illness in order to help to reduce smoking and to develop well-organised systems for monitoring hypertension and prescribing appropriate medication. One set of evidence is derived qualitatively from patients and requires an understanding about meaning and illness. The other set of evidence is derived quantitatively from controlled trials on effective treatment protocols for hypertension. It is possible to suggest that bringing these two sets of evidence together and providing a service that is competent in combining both sets of evidence is perhaps a precursor to understanding how to achieve an improvement in health outcome.

Over and above this, the management of activities of daily living and the positioning and handling of patients who have suffered from a stroke may be crucial in determining the degree of mobility and independence acquired by the patient following the stroke. Maintaining mobility and independence not only increases the quality of life for the patient, but also reduces care needs and demands for continuing care. However, as Pott recognises, this type of support needs to be integrated with existing patterns for managing activities of daily living, and, to make the limitations induced by the stroke acceptable, it has to link with the patient's own aspirations and goals in life.

In this context, data from Eurostat (Smedt, 1997) present an interesting picture of the situation in the European Community in 1994 prior to the inclusion of Austria, Finland and Sweden. These data demonstrate that almost 24 per cent of the European population reported being hampered in their daily activities by a chronic physical or mental health problem. This means that almost 66 million Europeans experience some degree of disability arising from the consequences of a chronic condition.

The impact of chronic disease on people's perceptions of their ability to manage their daily lives is, however, unevenly distributed across Europe. The impact of chronic disease on daily living activities is reported to be high in Portugal, the Netherlands and Germany, and relatively low in Spain, Ireland and Greece. This suggests that cultural interpretations of health and illness mediate people's responses to manifest disease processes. As van den Bos (1997) recognises, people with chronic diseases take up different positions in the continuum from health to illness and from independent to dependent living that may be unrelated to their manifest health needs arising from measures of physiological functioning. Identifying how people cope with disease processes and developing health care services that reflect these needs is important in developing models of appropriate health care intervention.

Health services are, therefore, faced with a complex agenda. Of paramount importance in contemporary government policy seems to be the desire to reduce hospital costs by increasing primary and community care services. Hospitals developed as centres of technical expertise; transferring this expertise into primary and community care, may not be cost-effective or even achievable. Primary care, therefore, needs to be about the twin problems of sustaining access to effective medical technology for those with continuing health care needs and addressing the phenomenological problem of understanding the patient's experience and meaning of symptoms and illness. It also needs to promote health in the face of disability by helping the patient and carers to address and overcome the daily limitations resulting from the disease process.

It is arguably the case that if these aspects of care are not understood and addressed, patients suffering from chronic, degenerative diseases are likely to make increasing demands for access to the new technologies in search of the elusive cure that will reintegrate them into society. These demands will be aided and abetted by the actions of primary health care workers in search of a similar solution to the patient's health problems (Pearson *et al.*, 1998).

Service changes that are designed to improve or control access to technology in either primary or secondary care, such as day surgery, or limiting prescribing, are likely to have the converse effect if the issue of meaning and the patient's daily experience of living with the illness are not addressed. Focusing on technological intervention may simply perpetuate and even increase the demand for that technology to compensate for addressing the deeper problem of overcoming self-stigma and learning to live effectively with the illness. Meeting the challenges raised by Pott (1992), described above, may be essential for addressing the government agenda of containing health care costs. Enabling patients to learn how to live with their illness may also enable them to identify the limitations of technology in managing their illness. Consequently, patients may only demand technology when they know that it can make a difference to their health.

Why then should health care professionals working in technologically advanced health care sectors address the remit derived from universal definitions of health? At one level, there is no reason why they should, other than the evidence of continued inequality and ideological and humanistic commitment. Arguably, universal health care policies are not in the interest of health care professionals. These policies require a fundamental change in culture from hierarchy to equality with currently marginalised and stigmatised groups, and the transfer of knowledge to these groups, to the detriment of the power and status currently vested in those who claim exclusive rights to this knowledge.

Some reasons, deriving from enlightened self-interest, can, however, be discerned for practitioners seeking to change their practice in line with the provision of care associated with universal definitions of health. The main self-interested reason is job satisfaction and the need to try to curtail the workload to an acceptable and effective level. Not addressing these issues will tend to perpetuate secondary and tertiary care at the expense of enabling patients to learn how to live a healthy life with their complex illnesses. Facilitating patients to live healthy lives may result in a reduced or better managed, less reactive demand for health care input over time, thus enabling health care professionals to spend more time with newly diagnosed or deteriorating patients and deal more effectively with the evolving workload.

If current trends in new technology and morbidity levels in an ageing population continue without addressing issues of expectation for health once ill, then debates about who has access to technology are likely to become more intense as demand increases and outstrips supply. Health care professionals will be caught in the centre of this squeeze and will become the front-line troops in implementing policies of health care rationing. They will frequently have to take tough, and what might appear to them, or to the patient, to be inequitable, decisions about who gets access to resources such as hospital beds on the basis of limited information in pressurised situations. Changing the way they work might ultimately be the only way in which health care professionals can keep their own stress down to an acceptable working level. As Maynard (1994) recognises, however, achieving this change is likely to be opposed by health care providers, in particular insurance companies and drug companies as well as some health care professionals, as it is unlikely to be in their long-term professional interest to pursue such approaches.

Selective approaches to provision	Universal approaches to provision
Serve the total population	Serve the total population
Assume an infinite demand for health care	Assume an infinite demand for health care
Provide access to technology based on professional assessment/rationing	Provide access to technology based on patient/professional assessment/ meaning
Patients gain access to technology on the basis of diagnosis and evidence that intervention is cost-effective	Aim to increase the knowledge and understanding of symptoms on the part of patient and health care professional(s)
	Rely on the patient to reduce his demand for technology based on a personal understanding of the symptoms plus an understanding of the effectiveness and limitations of the technology in managing the symptoms

Figure 3.2   Models of health care provision

It is possible to depict the dilemma facing health care professionals as a choice between two contrasting models of health care provision, as depicted in Figure 3.2.

Under the heading of selective approaches to health care provision, an increasing amount of health care work is focused on assessment to manage demand rather than intervention. Assessment is either labour intensive, requiring long interviews with the patient in order to elicit symptoms against a checklist of eligibility criteria, or technological in the form of laboratory tests, X-rays or CAT scans. These assessments are clearly vital in ensuring the application of an effective technology to a given set of symptoms. They become dysfunctional and costly when they are used as a basis for rationing access in the face of seemingly excessive demand.

In the selective model, infinite demand is managed through a rationing process that ideally, provides access to health care technology only to those patients exhibiting symptoms that can be treated cost-effectively. It excludes patients experiencing symptoms for which there is no diagnosis or cost-effective intervention. These patients (the volume of whom is currently unknown as they are difficult to record in a health information system based on codes for diagnosis) continue to make demands as their symptoms persist so are subject to an endless assessment process as this is the primary means of rationing access to effective health care technology.

A selective approach to health care provision conforms to the selective definitions of health described in the previous chapter. These include defining health as the absence of disease, maximising functional capacity, and improving psychosocial adjustment to circumstances, which can include adjusting the lifestyle to comply with medical instructions.

Universal approaches to health care provision are faced with the same set of population parameters, that is, infinite demand and a finite supply of cost-effective technology. A universal approach manages demand differently as it seeks to understand the patient's experience of health and illness, and locate the symptoms within these parameters. Those patients exhibiting symptoms indicative of diagnosable disease processes for which cost-effective technologies exist are given access to the technologies but are, more importantly, helped to understand when the technology is likely to be effective and comprehend the limitations of the technology in the context of their daily lifestyle. Patients can then moderate their demands for health care intervention based on a personal and knowledgeable understanding of the disease process and the efficacy of the technology in managing the disease process, rather than on repeated reassessment by professionals.

Those patients whose symptoms cannot be reduced by medical technology are not excluded from the system only to reappear, and be reassessed, as their symptoms persist. Instead, they are helped to gain a greater insight into their lifestyle and to adapt existing medical technologies in an attempt to manage their symptoms more effectively.

Both the selective and the universal approaches to health care provision are dealing with the same level of demand. Selective approaches attempt to manage demand through rationing processes that are themselves time-consuming and expensive. Universal approaches reject rationing as a basis for provision as this does not

---

Tier One:

Consists of non-specialist services delivered in a community setting. This level of service seeks ways of enabling all those coming into contact with children (teachers, parents, playworkers, dinner ladies) to recognise and manage difficult behaviour. This tier maintains a definition of such behaviour as normal childhood behaviour. In this way, it seeks to avoid the stigmatising effect of labelling such difficult behaviour as pathological

Tier Two:

This tier also operates in the community but provides access to multidisciplinary teams or individual practitioners with specialist skills in child and adolescent mental health. These services are provided on the basis that the targeted approach works better for higher-risk families and children when this approach is embedded within a universal programme that is itself embedded in the local community culture. Tier Two specialists supplement Tier One provision and practice within the arena of universal provision so that children experiencing mild problems but in need of specialist intervention are not singled out

Tier Three:

Consists of multiprofessional teams and out-patient services treating more severe disorders arising from psychological difficulties following physical, emotional or sexual abuse, severe family relationship problems or depression

Tier Four:

This tier is reserved for severe problems such as autism, in which the child and family might require access to specialist in-patient and out-patient services

---

Figure 3.3 Recommended tiers of service provision for child and adolescent mental health services

reduce demand but simply diverts it within the system, or postpones intervention to a later date when the problem has deteriorated sufficiently to warrant intervention. Universal approaches attempt to deal directly with demand by working with patients and their carers to reduce their dependency on health care technology and professional support. This is reflective of the definitions of health as independence, autonomy, growth and empowerment, which were described as universal definitions of health in the previous chapter.

If health care professionals seek to make an active, productive contribution to health rather than act as the main conduit for rationing, it is probable that this can only be achieved through the application of medical technology within a framework of universal approaches to health care provision. Two examples are given to illustrate the organisation of health care in which selective services are provided within a universal model of provision. These are described in Figures 3.3 and 3.4.

Figure 3.3 describes the four-tier arrangement for service provision recommended for child and adolescent mental health services (Health Advisory Service, 1995). This approach filters access to services according to the severity of the presenting condition. Children are only referred to tertiary services when less intensive sources of support are found to be ineffective or when a severe underlying condition such as autism is suspected. This reverses the current situation found in many areas, in which quite minor problems are referred directly to tertiary services for assessment and referred back to community services if they are available. In the absence of community services, children and adolescents with relatively minor problems are inappropriately treated at tertiary centres, or are only treated if the condition deteriorates sufficiently to warrant tertiary intervention. This creates long waiting lists on which children and adolescents with real and urgent needs are placed.

Figure 3.4 provides a diagrammatic representation of the recommended pathway for service provision for women suffering from urinary incontinence (Agency for Health Care Policy and Research, 1992; Royal College of Physicians, 1995). Female urinary incontinence is recognised to be a major problem for between 12 per cent and 20 per cent of the female population aged 45–64 years (Thomas *et al.*, 1980; Yarnell *et al.*, 1981; Holzt and Wilson, 1988). A range of first-line treatments, including pelvic floor exercises, vaginal cones, biofeedback techniques and neuromuscular electrical stimulation, are available and have been found to be effective (Agency for Health Care Policy and Research, 1992; Royal College of Physicians, 1995). Current guidelines recommend that all women suffering from this condition should be

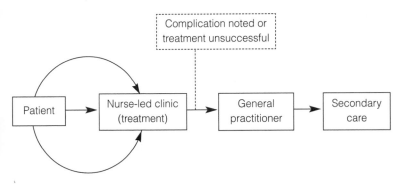

Figure 3.4 Recommended pathway for women accessing services for urinary incontinence

given access to first-line treatments prior to referral for secondary intervention (Agency for Health Care Policy and Research, 1992; Royal College of Physicians, 1995). Secondary intervention includes urodynamic studies to investigate the cause, as well as drugs and surgery.

However, as with child and adolescent services, first-line treatments are often not available, and women are either referred directly to secondary care or denied access to any form of service provision (Cheater, 1991; Knight and Procter, 1999). Concern about the ability of services to meet the high level of demand that would arise if first-line treatments were made more available acts to prevent primary care developments in this area (Knight *et al.*, 1999). This concern arises from the assumption that all treatments must be practitioner initiated, monitored and assessed. In fact, all first-line treatments have to be maintained by women at home. Making equipment available through chemists and other sources and educating women in its use may actually reduce the demand on services while simultaneously reducing the prevalence of this problem and even preventing deterioration requiring access to secondary interventions (Knight *et al.*, 1999).

In both child and adolescent mental health and the management of female urinary incontinence, there is evidence that, for many patients, primary and community-based services are not available. Patients are either denied access to services or referred to secondary and tertiary care in the first instance. Secondary providers then undertake a full assessment only to refer the patient back to primary care (if available), or inappropriately manage the problem through secondary or tertiary provision as primary and community-level services are not available. This massively increases the volume of patients accessing secondary and tertiary level services, making it difficult for these services to focus on those patients who would benefit most from this level of intervention.

Research into child and adolescent mental health and the management of female urinary incontinence suggests that a universal approach to health care provision may increase the effective use of medical technology by reducing referral within the system to this technology. In practice, this proposition is difficult to test, even in relation to the two services described above, as the conditions for universal provision are rarely available within health care systems based on selective principles. Considerable work, therefore, needs to be undertaken at the level of service provision to create the conditions in which to test the fundamental assumptions underpinning selective and universal approaches to health care provision in advanced industrial nations.

How should health care practitioners address the provision of universal health care?

One explanation consistently put forward for the continuation of inequality in both health care outcome and access to health services is the paradox that it is the middle classes who benefit most from the welfare state. They benefit not just as recipients, but also as providers. Health, social services and education provide stable jobs with good pensions, as well as free services when needed (Titmuss, 1958). This has given rise to what Tudor-Hart (1971) has termed the 'inverse care law', whereby those least in need receive more from public services (including jobs, job security and pensions, as well as access to the services) and consequently benefit more from their existence, while those with the greatest needs are marginalised and excluded.

From a social policy perspective, there are two ways in which the 'inverse care law' can be tackled. One way, perhaps the most effective, is to work towards a redistribution of wealth such that the discrepancy between wealthier and poorer sections of society is reduced. This is the approach advocated by Bradshaw (1994), who demonstrates that, in those countries where the gap between rich and poor has been narrowed, so too has the health gap. Income distribution is primarily the product of macro-economic policies, frequently outside the control of even national governments and subject to global economic forces. Within any nation state, however, economic policies can be pursued that aim to ameliorate the impact on the most disadvantaged sections of society of the consequences of turbulent global economic fortunes.

The health care industry is one of the biggest employees in Europe. Spending on health care in 1991 (expressed as a percentage of the gross domestic product) ranged from 5.2 in Greece, 6.6 in the UK, to 9.1 in France (Abel-Smith, 1994, p. 152). The recruitment and retention policies pursued specifically by nursing and more generally by health care could potentially be used to tackle some of the more enduring issues of exclusion and marginalisation experienced by disadvantaged sections of society. In this way, the health sector could work actively to redistribute income and life opportunities through its recruitment and employment strategies. The increasing amount of gross domestic product devoted to health care, whether publicly or privately, means that health care systems cannot be neutral to national and global economic forces. Whom health care systems recruit and how they educate and retain them will fundamentally affect issues associated with the distribution of income, security and life opportunities.

These policies impact at all levels within health care. They are fundamental to debates about recruitment to basic training, graduate status for nursing, equal opportunities, equal access to nursing and other health care professions, and training for disadvantaged people and those with disabilities. Academic lecturers, therefore, need to engage in these debates when developing their curricula and recruitment proforma. Higher education needs to consider the impact of institutional quality assurance indicators on enabling disadvantaged students to succeed and on encouraging lecturers to recruit such students. The NHS has to consider the merits of opening up recruitment opportunities and providing the flexible career structures that might be required if a broader range of people were to be successfully employed within this sector.

Nursing is the largest single occupational group within health care organisations (Keyzer, 1992). It has traditionally recruited from the constant supply of female school-leavers across all social classes (White, 1985). As Keyzer (1992) points out, this source is shrinking as other opportunities become available to female school-leavers. In response to this, nursing has recommended a widening of the entry gate to professional nurse education and the recruitment of mature men and women to nurse education programmes (UKCC, 1986). More recently, the need to open up pathways for support workers into nurse education has also been acknowledged (DoH, 1999).

The need to maintain such a large workforce has challenged nursing to strive continuously for new ways in which to open up recruitment opportunities in health care. Consequently, nursing is well placed, strategically, to link in with diverse population groups. This puts nursing in a good position to address structurally some of the issues associated with inequality in health, described above. In the past, the wide social class entry into nursing has been viewed as problematic. Nurses were seen simultaneously to pursue both professionalising strategies associated with the recruitment of nurses from middle-class families, and trade union worker/manager strategies associated with nurses who viewed nursing as an occupation rather than a profession (White, 1985). In the context of addressing inequalities in health, however, this wide recruitment becomes advantageous as pathways are made available for relatively disadvantaged and disenfranchised sections of the population to gain the necessary academic and work experience to enter nurse training. It must also be recognised, however, that there are still barriers to advancement for disadvantaged groups, particularly indigenous ethnic minority groups in the UK, to gain entry to nursing, and further work needs to be undertaken to understand and, where appropriate, overcome these barriers.

Another, more targeted approach that lies within the remit of health and social care practitioners is to recognise and compensate for inequality in health by introducing services designed to meet the specific needs of disadvantaged or vulnerable populations. Flaskerud and Winslow define vulnerable populations as 'social groups who experience limited resources and consequently high relative risk for morbidity and premature mortality' (Flaskerud and Winslow, 1998, p. 69). In developing services targeted at vulnerable populations, it may be necessary to adapt the way in which they are delivered or to provide additional support to ensure that these services can be effectively utilised and the benefits maintained over time.

The examples of child and adolescent mental health services and the management of female urinary incontinence given above represent two very different health care problems. As the examples illustrate, however, thinking about provision in new ways opens up access to services for disadvantaged groups of patients whose problems are currently neglected within contemporary forms of service provision. By adopting a universal approach, resources can be redistributed in order to increase the number of people able to access services, without necessarily requiring additional resources. It does, however, require a redistribution of the way in which existing resources are used and service priorities identified. It also needs a sharing of expertise and a shift in provision from expert/specialist practitioner to knowledgeable/generalist practitioner, and the sharing of knowledge openly and freely with patients and their families.

The contribution of nursing to developing universal services

Much of nursing theory and work is concerned with maintaining activities of daily living within the everyday lives of people suffering from either enduring disabilities or temporary disruptions arising from acute episodes and/or interventions. In practice, nurses take account of the physiological parameters of a person's health but are more concerned with the daily management of the symptoms than with seeking a cure. As a result, their work entails confronting the consequences for patients' lives and for their families arising from the condition, and helping patients and families to manage their condition effectively. This is recognised by Borst-Eilers, Minister for Health, Welfare and Sport in the Netherlands, who suggests that:

> caring for the chronically ill involves what one might describe as the core business of nursing... According to the textbooks nursing is about supporting, restoring or taking over activities which people temporarily or permanently cannot perform for themselves. Unlike doctors, nurses and carers do not concern themselves with the causes of illness, but with its implications. Where the chronically ill are concerned, those implications are persistent; such people must learn how to live with their condition. (Borst-Eilers, 1997, p. 3)

In this context, Grundy's (1997) discussion of the evidence of a reduction in the extent of serious disability and a marked drop in the proportion of people unable to undertake four activities of daily living without assistance may form the basis of developing outcome indicators that reflect nursing contributions to health. Grundy attributes much of this reduction to the recognition of the disabling consequences of bedrest. Bedrest is an activity that for many years provided the core focus for nursing care. It is possible that the way in which nursing care is delivered could have a profound effect on the extent to which people are able to maintain independence in the face of a deteriorating chronic condition and on the demands they make over time for support with daily activities of living. Keeping people independent is the key to managing demand for nursing, which in itself forms the single biggest health professional group in the UK.

Interestingly, nursing has developed a research tradition dominated by, and in many cases derived from, qualitative, interactionist and phenomenological perspectives. It is these research perspectives which are best placed to deal with issues of the meaning and contextualisation of the illness in terms of the social and psychological fabric of the patient's life. As discussed above by Pott (1992, p. xiv), 'the chronically ill person has to learn to accept the illness'. Learning to accept the illness is probably the single biggest hurdle that people suffering from chronic diseases have to overcome. It is also one of the most neglected aspects of our current health care provision. This aspect of health care is unlikely to be developed using quantitative research traditions that focus on achieving standardisation rather than understanding diversity. The now well-established qualitative research traditions in nursing could, if their value were appreciated, make a major contribution to developing evidence-based services that enable patients to learn how to live full and healthy lives in the face of degenerating illness.

Summary and conclusion

This chapter has provided an empirical foundation for the adoption of universal approaches to health care provision. The case for universal provision rests on the combined effect of social, psychological, cultural and environmental experiences in determining life expectancy and experiences of illness in later life. Such factors also impact on the way in which the patient deals with illness once it arises. Second, the vast majority of illness and disability in advanced industrial nations is chronic and degenerative. Managing this type of illness requires universal definitions of health that promote autonomy, independence, self-determination, empowerment and social inclusion, rather than the more passive and socially isolating definitions associated with selective definitions of health.

In the context of chronic illness, selective definitions of health are difficult to sustain as these definitions require health professionals continuously to reassess patient access to health technology. Consequently, selective approaches divert professional activity away from delivering effective interventions towards undertaking increasing amounts of assessment, which acts as the main conduit for rationing within a selective system. In a population that is unlikely to be cured and so is unlikely to realise discharge from the service, this approach has a tendency to increase dependency as the disease progresses. In contrast, health care provision based on universal definitions of health ensures that each encounter between a patient and health care worker is productive in the sense that it seeks to promote autonomy and independence from service provision. This is undertaken within a framework that acknowledges the enduring and frequently deteriorating health care needs of the patient.

Contemporary approaches to health care provision are, however, highly selective and reflective of the biomedical model that dominates selective definitions of health. Nursing, health visiting and social work have, however, developed theories and models of practice based on universal definitions of health as autonomy and empowerment. An exploration of these models may well provide a framework for understanding how health care systems can move from provision based on selectivity to encompass the universal definitions of health enshrined in contemporary health care policy. The remainder of this book looks at the role of nursing in taking on this remit.

Chapter 4

Caring for Health

The previous chapter described present and predicted trends in the incidence of illness and disability across the Western population. It illustrated how improved social conditions have given rise to an increase in life expectancy and the concentration of disability towards the end of the lifespan. However, although people are living longer, they are also more sick for increasing lengths of time (Bebbington, 1991). As yet, material improvements have not resulted in a reduction in the number of disability-free years across the whole population.

Access to health care is predominantly selective based on the presence of symptoms. Health care providers, therefore, tend to have an effect once the disease process has become established. Given this scenario, the need to further develop health care interventions to minimise the level of disability and dependency arising from disease processes seems to be essential. Such an approach could include the universal definitions of health discussed in Chapter 2, such as 'growth', 'autonomy', 'self-determination' and 'well-being'. These are equally as applicable to individuals who have succumbed to illness and to those who care for them, as they are to those not yet experiencing ill-health.

The term 'health care' is commonly used to describe the work of the health services. The previous two chapters have concentrated on the concept of health; this chapter focuses on the concept of care. It begins with a discussion of the theoretical literature on caring. It discusses the role of nursing within the context of the caring literature, illustrating the links between nursing work and the family caring work traditionally ascribed to women. It ends by presenting an analysis of the impact of caring on the lives of carers, as depicted in the social policy literature. The chapter reviews the role of nursing and social care provision in both sustaining and determining the role of family carers, who in turn sustain the health of families.

Caring and nursing

Care as a concept and as a practice is elusive and difficult to define, much of this difficulty deriving from its universal appeal as a defining feature of humanity. Brykczynska (1997), in a review of the literature on caring, suggests that, at a philosophical level, caring is frequently characterised as a moral obligation and a human imperative. It is incumbent on people to care for others, and to do so defines their humanness. It is also depicted as an ethical way of being, which results from moral development. Here, people understand the value of caring and use the principles of caring to guide their behaviour.

Burnard (1997) views caring as an almost universal phenomenon, one that is linked to the very process of becoming and being a person. Morse *et al.* (1991, p. 122), commenting on theories that define caring as a human trait, suggest that 'caring is generally perceived to be a basic constant characteristic that forms the foundation of human society. Caring is considered necessary for human survival – an essential component of being human.'

Definitions of caring such as those given by Burnard (1997) and described by Morse *et al.* (1991) indicate that caring is frequently viewed as a universal and fundamental activity; consequently, it is difficult to claim caring as the province of any one professional group or organisation. Caring is what defines our humanity. It follows that it is an activity engaged in by everyone who claims to contribute to social well-being.

In health care, however, caring work is frequently identified as the focus of nursing practice (Watson, 1985; Leininger, 1988). This is not to say that other professions do not engage in caring work but merely to recognise that nursing, more perhaps than any other profession, has claimed caring as its province. In nursing, caring is increasingly being linked to concepts of 'humanness' and 'being', as depicted in the work of phenomenologists such as Husserl and Heidegger.

For Benner and Wrubel (1989), who adopt a phenomenological perspective, caring is fundamentally about values. It is about the things (people, projects and events) that really matter to us. Caring is simultaneously about 'being connected... it fuses thought, feeling, and action – knowing and being' and about 'differentiating' (Benner and Wrubel, 1989, p. 1). Through caring we know what we value, what we wish to be connected with or to. Equally importantly, through caring, which 'fuses thought, feeling, and action', we are able to identify those things which are *less* important to us – we are able to *differentiate*, to identify our priorities. Caring not only tells us what is important in our lives, but also tells us what is less important to us. Here again, caring has a universal quality, enabling us to chart a course through life by attending to the things we value most.

In developing an analysis of caring in nursing, Brykczynska (1992) has explored the five attributes of caring first identified by Roach (1985). These are compassion, confidence, competence, conscience and commitment, which are described as core to operationalising caring in nursing. Roach places great emphasis on the development of caring relationships and the responsibilities that such relationships entail. In developing her theory of caring, Roach links effective caring relationships to concepts of growth and self-actualisation, suggesting that caring can evoke developmental relationships. For Roach, then, caring encompasses universal definitions of health associated with growth and self-actualisation, as described in Chapter 2.

Morse *et al.* (1991), in a review of conceptualisations of caring in the nursing literature, identify five conceptualisations of caring:

1. *caring as a human trait,* in which caring is described as being part of human nature, common to and inherent in all people;

2. *caring as a moral imperative,* caring being viewed as a moral virtue that promotes human dignity and respect for patients as people;

3. *caring as an effect,* which recognises the emotional dimension to caring in which feelings of compassion and empathy are evoked, these motivating the nurse to provide care for the patient;

4. *caring as an interpersonal interaction,* in which caring is viewed as a mutual endeavour between the nurse and the patient, both parties being communicative, trustful, respected and committed to each other;

5. *caring as a therapeutic intervention,* the nurse identifying and meeting the patient's needs for care regardless of how the nurse feels; caring is viewed as a skilled activity and caring competencies are identified.

Morse *et al.* identify three outcomes of caring: the patient's subjective experience, the patient's physical response and the nurse's subjective experience.

The nursing literature acknowledges the universal nature of caring but seeks to identify the professional competencies associated with caring as a professional endeavour. Emphasis is placed on the development of relationships through which caring work evolves and takes effect. The interactive nature of the caring relationship between the nurse and the patient is acknowledged. The need to strive towards universal definitions of health, such as growth and self-actualisation, as well as dignity and maintaining human integrity is frequently discussed.

Caring and social policy

Bulmer has depicted care as having three components:

> (1) physical tending, which is the most intimate kind; (2) material and psychological support which does not involve physical contact; and (3) more generalised concern about the welfare of others, which may or may not lead to the other two types of help. Superimposed upon this three-fold distinction is a further distinction between 'care as labour' and 'care as communal action. (Bulmer, 1987, p. 21)

The distinction between 'care as labour' and 'care as communal action' is pervasive in social policy literature and reflects a concern (or care) to support but not invade areas of life that are considered to be private. In the UK, the Seebohm Report (DHSS, 1968), for example, encouraged social services departments to work as part of a network of formal and informal support, co-ordinating services and mobilising community resources, in particular volunteers, to meet identified needs. Bulmer (1987) discusses the delicate relationship that exists between formal and informal carers and the importance of inter-weaving service provision with informal care while simultaneously not undermining the family's and local community's capacity to respond to the needs of its members. For Bulmer, family care and informal local care are sacrosanct, while the role of health and social care organisations is supportive and redistributive.

In practice, however, as Bulmer notes, the concept of health and social care provision as supportive of and even subservient to family and informal care is belied by the relative status attached to each set of activities. Formal care provided through health and social care organisations operates in the public domain. These organisations receive public funding, are subject to public scrutiny and provide a vehicle for the development of professional careers, which are, in some cases, highly prestigious and coveted. Research is increasingly forming an integral part of formal care provision, the more established health care professions claiming status by defining a circumscribed, research-based body of knowledge that underpins their practice.

Family and informal care on the other hand, while highly valued, receive minimal financial reward, are frequently costly for the family (Le Grand, 1982) and impact negatively on the opportunity for predominantly female family members to pursue individual and autonomous personal goals (Pond and Popay, 1983). Moreover, because family and informal care reside outside the public domain, opportunities to research family care are negligible, and the care is viewed as individually and culturally determined.

The status distinction between formal and informal care is reflected in a similar status distinction between 'care as communal action' and 'care as labour'. Here, the more generalised redistributive and supportive functions and treatments provided by health and social care associated with communal action have been legitimised as areas of public concern, debate, research, policy initiative and investment. The media, for example, frequently reports on breakthroughs in new medical technology, while the issue of care in the community is endlessly debated and reformulated in policy initiatives such as HAZs (DoH, 1998a) and the Healthy Living Centres initiative in the UK (DoH, 1998b).

The intimate aspects of 'care as labour' or tending provided by families, nurses, nursery nurses, childminders, nannies and residential care workers, and the emotional labour (Smith, 1992) of individual psychological and social support mechanisms associated with care as labour, remain, however, private and obscure. Lawler (1991), in an anthropological study of hospital nursing in Australia, highlights how the intimate work undertaken by nurses providing physical care for patients breaks social taboos, rendering such work secret. It is generally avoided as an unsocial topic by those not directly engaged in it and is, therefore, difficult to publicise or scrutinise. A similar point is made by Smith and Agard (1997); referring to the work of a public health nurse in the USA, they comment, 'Despite the title of *public*-health nurse, much of the "public" is unaware of the work she does' (Smith and Agard, 1997, p. 183, original emphasis). The activities of physical and emotional care associated with nursing, therefore, locate it within the sphere of 'care as labour', a sphere normally seen as the province of families and outside the domain of public provision.

It is here that many of the most difficult ethical and moral dilemmas of service provision are located. They are difficult because, rather than there being a continuum from formal to informal care within which the intimate care associated with nursing could be located, a number of writers have suggested that the two forms of care (formal and informal) are fundamentally incompatible. Bulmer (1987) relates this to the distinction made by Max Weber between bureaucratic modes of action, which are governed by a rational-legal authority, and affective modes of action, which are governed by traditional authority and characterised by feelings and emotions. Consequently, the interface between formal and informal care is recognised as being 'fraught with discontinuities and contradictions in its underlying assumptions and features' (Froland, 1980, p. 574).

Abrams (1980) has proposed that the rules and assumptions governing bureaucratically administered services are the antithesis of the norms and relationships that drive informal caring networks. This analysis suggests that the more authority the organisation invests in legal and rational decision-making processes, the more difficult it is for those working at the interface of formal and informal care to accomplish the task of interweaving the affective domain of care with the formal structures of service provision.

Lipsky (1991) explores this problem in his analysis of the distribution of social security payments in the USA. Lipsky describes how, in the 'implementation of social welfare programmes there remains an irreducible extent to which worker discretion cannot be eradicated' (Lipsky, 1991, p. 212). In other words, if social security payments are to be effective in responding to individual circumstances, some degree of worker discretion in the allocation of payments is essential. Worker discretion enables payments to remain sensitive and responsive to individual needs and reduces the impact on individuals of an overly bureaucratic approach to payments, which dictates eligibility independently of any knowledge or understanding of their circumstances. Lipsky's work highlights how worker discretion in managing the interface between social welfare systems and individual circumstances is likely to increase as single bureaucratic solutions have been found to be both ineffective and insensitive to the complex and multidimensional needs arising from individual circumstances.

A similar dilemma has been identified by Coyne (1995) in his discussion of professional interventions in family relationships to improve family coping with illness, which he suggests remains a 'neglected edge' in professional efforts to improve dealing with illness. Coyne argues for the development of a more systematic approach to interventions in family relationships in order to facilitate controlled outcome studies. He suggests that qualitative case examples cannot justify routine intervention by professionals in family relationships. He recognises, however, that the current practice of excluding spouses and family members from routine involvement in health care while simultaneously assuming that they will meet the demands of coping without assistance can neither be justified nor sustained.

While Bulmer (1987) emphasises the sanctity of privacy in conducting family affairs free from interference from outside agencies, Gould (1984) highlights the numerous ways in which the state intrudes into personal lives through the legislation, customs and traditions associated with marriage. Despite more liberal interpretations, Gould argues that it is still the case that the marriage contract is legally interpreted primarily using the traditional model of gender roles and responsibilities. Women are still expected to perform their caring role in the family as unpaid labour, and this devalues the contribution of women's work in the economy at large. James (1994) highlights how the welfare legislation arising from the Beveridge Report assumed female dependency on male breadwinners and placed an obligation on family members to care for each other, assuming throughout that everyone lived in families. Gould argues that the separation between the public and private spheres should in fact be more distinct than it is at present and that personal relationships should be deinstitutionalised.

The above literature highlights the complexity surrounding caring work. On the one hand it is considered a universal human attribute, but on the other there is a concern not to interfere with the caring work carried out by families. Policies to support caring work do so within a legislative and policy framework that is imbued with assumptions about gender roles, responsibilities and rewards, while at the same time claiming neutrality. Caring work itself cuts across both public and private spheres of provision, while some aspects of caring work, particularly in health care, have been professionalised and carry considerable economic reward and social prestige.

Caring as women's work

Whitbeck (1984, p. 82), in a critique of mainstream approaches to philosophy and ethics, outlines what she considers to be a core human *practice*, that is, 'the mutual realisation of people, sometimes described as nurturing'. According to Whitbeck, the concept of mutual realisation recognises that 'One becomes a person in and through relationships with other people; being a person requires that one has a history of relationships with other people, and the realisation of the self can be achieved only in and through relationships and practices'. Whitbeck lists among the forms of this work the rearing of children, the education of children and adolescents, the care of the dying, the nursing of the sick and injured, and a variety of spiritual practices related to daily life. These activities are distinguished by their recognition that all parties to the relationship and participants in the practice emerge and develop, and, therefore, the relationships and practices also develop.

Furthermore, in pursuing this practice, not only are certain ends achieved, but also it creates certain ways of living and develops certain characteristics (virtues) in those who participate and try to achieve standards of excellence in this practice. In other words, it creates a culture of care by which this core practice is learnt and passed on to others. This reflects the definitions of caring as a universal human trait described earlier and Burnard's definition of caring as the very process of becoming and being a person.

Whitbeck recognises that the practice of mutual realisation can take a variety of forms, most if not all of which are regarded as women's work. Consequently, she argues that mainstream philosophers and ethicists have largely ignored this practice, marginalising an activity that is arguably fundamental to a comprehensive analysis of human development.

Graham (1984), using an entirely different literature, draws a similar conclusion about the marginalisation of women's work in mainstream political and academic thought. Graham was concerned to explore the link between social and structural inequalities and the capacity of families to fulfil their role in health maintenance. She asks the question, 'What are the sources of support on which families depend for their survival?', highlighting three fundamental forms of support: women's care, the family income over which women have control and the external provision of goods and services. Graham cites evidence to suggest that, despite their increasing involvement in the labour market, women continue to meet the health needs of their partners and children. These needs are not only the needs arising from illness or a breakdown in health, but more importantly derive from the daily activities necessary to sustain family health: shopping, cooking and paying the bills.

It follows that, in most households, the health-sustaining income is the income controlled by the mother. Graham describes women's income as a vital determinant of family welfare, providing the resources necessary to sustain family health. The income that women control is determined in part by the labour market and in part by relations within the family. While a considerable amount of research has been conducted into the public domain of the labour market, very little is known about how income is distributed within the private sphere of families, yet this may crucially determine family access to the resources necessary to sustain health. Consequently, Graham suggests, women are often left to juggle two paradoxical demands: the demand for income in order to purchase the resources necessary for health, such as food, shelter, warmth and leisure, and the demands of those being cared for, for her presence to nurture and sustain their daily development.

Graham also describes how family health requires a social environment conducive to health maintenance. Access to clean air, quality housing, transport, leisure, shopping and play facilities is crucial in enabling families to maintain health. Poverty, when combined with poor housing and poor transport facilities, severely curtails the extent to which families can make use of the health or leisure facilities necessary to maintain their physical and mental health. In discussing the literature on the role of families in maintaining health, Graham comments that:

> the maintenance of family health is the least well-documented area of lay health care. Despite the popular and political interest in the family, we know very little about the physical and psychological labour of sustaining human life. While the family is recognised to be Britain's primary and most important health care institution, we remain surprisingly ignorant about how it works. (Graham, 1984, p. 153)

The analyses given by Whitbeck (1984) and Graham (1984), although deriving from widely different sources of literature, highlight the tendency in mainstream academic writing to focus on the public domain. The private domain of women's work is dismissed as being too emotionally unstable to contribute to developing academic knowledge, or too personal to allow the imposition of essentially public goals such as health and education to be attributed directly to the daily activities of family members. Thus, as Graham's work demonstrates, a thorough analysis of the resources required by women to sustain family health has yet to be undertaken, and women are expected to cope with the circumstances as they find them. So what are the parallels between family care and nursing, and what can be gained by studying them? A number of parallels are described below and the implications for research and practice discussed.

24-hour care

The most obvious parallel between nursing and family care is that both provide 24-hour care in the form of actually ensuring continuity of care for the person(s) being cared for. Like family carers, nurses are the primary carers in health care institutions. Family care is characterised as being unpaid and based in the home, where it becomes a 24-hour 'on-call' responsibility (James, 1992). A carer can only be freed from caring responsibilities when alternative caring arrangements can be made. These take numerous forms: other family members, friends, nursery, childminders, schools and day centres, for example. Some, such as schools, are statutory, others have to be organised by the carer, and some have to be paid for. Like carers, a nurse can only go 'off duty' when the next carer/nurse arrives. A carer's life is, therefore, circumscribed by the alternative arrangements made for caring. A failure in these arrangements, for whatever reason, pulls carers back into their caring role or prevents them leaving it.

There is also a degree of reciprocity in these arrangements even when they are paid for. Respect for each other's responsibilities means that the secondary carer has to arrive on time and the primary carer has to return on time. The delicate balance of care arrangements is severely disrupted if either party abuses or exploits the situation, by, for example, working late and not returning on time. Shift handovers in nursing are similarly characterised by the same recognition of reciprocity. In order not to be kept late at work, nurses tend to avoid turning up late for shifts as to turn up late keeps another nurse on duty.

The notion of reciprocity between carers is an important feature of caring work and one worthy of further study in relation to the organisation and management of this type of work (Nolan *et al.*, 1996). It is quite probably a feature of the style of 'coping management' described by Davies (1992) but possibly not one that has been recognised, valued and researched. The potential contribution that an understanding of the concept of reciprocity between carers could make to the organisation of nursing will be discussed further in the Chapter 5.

But what is caring for? The discussion earlier highlighted its universal nature and moral worth. Such lofty attributes are, however, difficult to identify as a basis for daily activity. Benner and Wrubel (1989) defined caring as connecting thought, feeling and action in order to identify *what matters*. The objects of care, namely their families, clearly matter to the individuals who stay at home and care for them. However, despite the essentially privatised nature of family care, there is an increasing body of knowledge that links the way in which people are cared for with their physical and psychological growth and development.

Caring routines

Graham (1984) describes how work for health in families is achieved through the patterning of the day. The fragile equilibrium created by the need to meet the 24-hour demands of family members becomes embedded in routines that are designed to maximise the restricted flexibility of the carer's daily life. These routines encompass aspects of daily living such mealtimes, bedtime routines and punctuality for school and work. Important aspects of physical, psychological and social health, including nutrition, time keeping, sleeping, leisure and exercise are embedded within these routines. Graham describes how aspects of daily living that give rise to conflict, such as taking children shopping, are often managed by a recourse to apparently unhealthy behaviours such as providing sweets in order to achieve the goal of family harmony. These routines remain fairly stable over prolonged periods of time and limit opportunities for choice and the exercise of responsibility, which, as Graham highlights, provides a focus for much health promotion literature.

Graham's work highlights the way in which routines are used by families to resolve enduring conflicts that arise in accomplishing the many different tasks required to sustain health, to provide 24-hour care and to harmonise the competing demands of family members. She suggests that 'Caring is about reconciling as well as meeting commitments; it is about containing demands and conserving supplies to ensure that needs and ends meet' (Graham, 1984, p. 152). Graham's work illustrates how the resources at the disposal of the family influence the family routine, prioritise needs and resolve conflicts and demands in more or less healthy ways. Routines determine the parameters of choice in lifestyle available to families at any single point in time, but are also deeply flexible as they mould to the changing circumstances and fortunes of the family and the developing needs of the offspring.

Routines are similarly used in nursing to manage the daily demands made by patients and to resolve the enduring conflicts that arise in accomplishing the many different tasks required to provide patient care (Alaszewski, 1977; Procter, 1989a). Routines are used to demarcate the workload and to prioritise between the different and competing needs of patients for nursing care. As in family care, the nursing routine shapes the therapeutic environment, moulding to the daily exigencies arising from the unpredictable nature of patient care. Routines determine the organisation of the patient's day, the ways in which care is delivered and the therapeutic outcomes embedded in the delivery of care: dignity, respect, individualised and responsive help, standardised provision, health promotion, independence or dependency.

As with family routines, routines in nursing are also reflective of the resources available to care and the organisation of these resources to meet patient care needs. Through routines, nurses seek to circumscribe patient demand to that which can be met by the supply and skill of regularly available nursing staff (Procter, 1989a). Nurses seek to constrain demand via the routine and to stabilise the supply and skill mix of nurses in order to ensure that needs and ends meet. In the practice of 'care as labour', as against abstract philosophical theories of care, both family carers and nurses confront the universal and abstract moral imperatives of caring by imposing boundaries on their caring work through the development of caring routines.

The extent to which these routines promote health, well-being and quality of life for all participants in the relationship appears largely to depend on the level of resource available to the carers. According to Graham's analysis, in family health the income over which women have control appears to be a crucial determinant of health-promoting family routines. In health care, the nursing resource and skill mix may be fundamental to developing health-promoting routines in hospital and other institutional settings. Most of the literature on skill mix in nursing currently focuses on tasks accomplished rather than the outcomes embedded in the daily routine and the skill and supply of nursing and other resources that determines that routine. This issue is discussed more fully in Chapter 7.

Caring contradictions

While family care is frequently considered sacrosanct and not subject to public scrutiny, the concept of caring in nursing has similarly been considered a worthy end, not subject to critical debate (Morse *et al.*, 1991). There is, however, a growing body of literature that testifies to the foundation of much psychological and physical ill-health in family relationship and behaviour patterns (Bowlby, 1969, 1973, 1980; Miller, 1995). Winnicott (1960) recognised that children and parents exist in relationship to each other. There is a feedback loop whereby the feelings and behaviours of one affect the feelings and behaviours of the other, each cycle of feedback modifying the way in which each party participates in the relationship. Blaxter (1981, p. 150), in a discussion of models of child–adult relationships, has noted the 'self-righting and

self-organising tendency' found in children, which moves them towards
normality even when faced with pressures towards deviation. Here, it is
suggested that children are active in organising their world and responsive to the processes embedded in their daily transactions with others.

In reviewing this literature, Reder and Lucey (1995) identify the
importance of the attachment dynamic, described by Bowlby, as being
particularly significant; in this, the provision of a secure emotional
base in early life facilitates the development of self-esteem, a capacity
for autonomous functioning and empathy for others, key characteristics associated with the universal definitions of health described in
Chapter 2. Reder and Lucey (1995, p. 6) conclude:

> There is now general consensus that child maltreatment is the end-result of
> interplay between predisposed caretakers who are caught in conflictual
> relationship patterns, vulnerable children and external stressors, with no
> single factor 'causing' the abusive behaviour. Parents, or other primary
> caretakers, carry into adult life unresolved residues of adverse childhood
> experiences which may intrude into their relationship with partners and
> with their own children and can be exaggerated by social stress.

The literature on caring described above also highlighted the importance of relationships in achieving caring in practice. However, the
literature remained ambivalent on the role of the patient in shaping the
relationship. It also adopted an idealised stance, which assumes that
nurses are themselves free from unresolved residues of childhood experiences and are able to develop caring relationships unimpeded by social
and psychological stressors.

In contrast, it is possible to suggest that the interactive and potentially
conflictual nature of family caring is paralleled in nursing in relation to
definitions of 'good' and 'bad' patients. There is a substantive nursing literature on the unpopular patient. Kelly and May (1982), in a review of this
literature, recognise that the good patient is frequently the conforming
patient. They argue, however, for an interactionist approach to studying
manifestations of popular and unpopular patients, suggesting that:

> Patients... are not passive recipients of nursing labels... As parties to the
> interaction they retain power to influence, shape, and ultimately reject
> nurses' attempts to impose their definition of the situation, with profound
> consequences for nurse–patient relations, and by extension for the nursing
> task itself. (Kelly and May, p. 154)

In the course of this argument, Kelly and May suggest that nurses
'symbolically take the role of patient both to make, and to make sense

of their own role, and it is in so doing that the labelling of patients inevitably takes place. The good patient is one who conforms to the role of the nurse: the bad patient denies that legitimation' (Kelly and May, p. 154). Like children, patients are proactive in shaping and responding to the care environment, but, like children, they risk being labelled 'unpopular' if they stray too far from the behaviour deemed appropriate by their carers.

In recognition of the proactivity of patients in responding to the care environment, Thorne and Robinson (1989) have described the evolution of relationships between health care practitioners and patients suffering from chronic illness as being characterised by 'guarded alliance'. Guarded alliance is the patients' response to the degree to which they feel able to trust a health care professional, this in turn being influenced by the degree of confidence the professional feels in the patients' and families' own competence to manage the illness effectively. Thorne and Robinson recognise that, in the real world of health care, caring relationships, such as those described in the nursing literature, are rare and difficult to achieve. Professionals do not always trust patients and are not always able to develop the attributes of confidence, commitment, competence, compassion and conscience identified by Roach (1985) as being characteristic of effective caring.

Caring can, therefore, give rise to paradoxical outcomes. The intensity and/or enduring nature of the relationship provides an environment characterised by compromise and negotiation between competing needs, including those of the care giver. Routines manage the demands and absorb conflicts. Routines evolve slowly over time, and the interplay between the different parties involved embeds behavioural patterns in the routine. This process may or may not promote health, well-being or quality of life for any or all of the participants.

The interactionist perspective advocated by Kelly and May (1982) clearly goes some way towards explaining the labelling of patients that takes place in nursing. However, as with family care, good nursing care needs to understand how routines evolve from the predisposing characteristics and experiences bought to the situation by all parties and the interactive nature of the environment for care work. Together, these create the 'culture of care' described by Whitbeck (1984), through which the core practice of caring is learnt and passed on to others. In developing an understanding of this core practice, carer/recipient characteristics and behaviours, as well as the routines of practice that evolve from them, need to be analysed without demanding compliant behaviour from either party.

Compliance: a moral imperative

A further parallel between nursing and women's work arises out of the consequences for each party of the interactive relationship. Moral judgements about the appropriate behaviour of the child, the patient and the carer create a coercive environment in which both nursing and family care take place. Compliant behaviour in children is frequently seen to be a sign of good parenting. Acknowledging a child's frustrations by allowing him to scream endlessly in the supermarket is severely frowned upon, despite the appropriateness of the child's reaction to the situation. Carers either do not take the child shopping or control this behaviour. As Graham (1984) demonstrates with regard to sweets, parents frequently use bribes and other seemingly unhealthy behaviours in order to appear in public settings to have well-behaved children.

Similarly, patients whose fears and anxieties are not 'under control' at the time of treatment and investigation are also frowned upon, as it can hold the process up and interfere with scheduling. Nurses, like family carers, clearly have a duty to manage the emotional environment in order to ensure that appropriate behaviour is displayed by patients at appropriate times (Smith, 1992). Fears and anxieties must be displaced to more convenient times, such as the middle of the night, when they will not interfere with treatment or, in the case of children, shopping or schooling. The moral imperative to appear to be coping, regardless of the personal cost, appears as a recurrent theme in the practice of care-as-labour, upheld by both carer and those being cared for alike.

Baker's (1983) research into nursing on a care of the elderly ward demonstrates how the organisational and cultural processes of the hospital converge to label nursing behaviour that addresses the emotional and psychological needs of patients at the time they arise as being disruptive of hospital teams and inefficient from an organisational perspective. Baker's work demonstrates how patient-centred nursing on the part of one ward sister (Sister Green) gave rise to complaints of alleged inefficiency from medical staff and hospital managers. If patient-centred styles of nursing are viewed as inefficient by authority figures in the hospital, they are unlikely to be adopted by nurses who are usually considered to be junior to medical staff and managers, and relatively low paid in comparison with these staff. Baker (1983, p. 114) states that:

> it is interesting to note that Sister Green's [style of nursing], which appeared to be unacceptable to everyone but the patients, seemed more

closely than its alternative, to approximate to the recommendations of nurse leaders and nursing literature... [and] accorded with the recommendations of official [Department of Health and Social Security] policy.

Baker's work reinforces the congruence between nursing and the wider health care policy agenda but illustrates a failure on the part of hospitals to create environments in which caring routines that seek to address psychological and emotional needs, necessary to meet these policy objectives, can flourish.

By locating emotional work in the home and family, workplaces are enabled to pursue rational organisational goals, unimpeded by the problems and difficulties of dealing with people's emotions (Anthony, 1977). When it is transferred into organisational settings, emotional work is usually undertaken by the lowest and least powerful grades of staff, who carry this work out unobtrusively, ensuring that it does not intrude into the mainstream activities of the organisation. James (1992) demonstrates the transferability of skills learnt in the domestic arena into workplace settings in order to manage the emotional components of caring for terminally ill patients in a hospice. In her study, James found that auxiliaries most frequently undertook this work because it was time-consuming and required a considerable knowledge of the patient as a person. The ready availability of auxiliaries and close physical contact offered a regular opportunity for effective emotional labour.

The above, very brief, review of the complex interactive nature of nursing and family care highlights how paying attention to the detailed emotional needs of patients and family members can create a disruption of the smooth running of an organisation. The pursuit of technical and rational efficiency sets up a coercive environment in which nurses and patients, parents and children, have to manage emotional behaviour in order to be seen as being effective in their role. This is reflected in the work of James (1992, p. 503), who concludes:

> In hospital care... and in some hospices, the needs of the organisation and physical care come first while the emotional labour remains largely informal and grafted on to the dominant biomedical, physical system.

For this to change, organisations/society need to understand emotional work in order to create an environment in which the mutual realisation described by Whitbeck (1984) as the core practice of women's work can be practised without coercion. As Whitbeck (1984, p. 81) points out:

The liberation of women's [and nurses'] relationships and practices requires that those practices and relationships be so reconstituted that the skills, sensitivities, and virtues, which make it possible for people to contribute to one another's development, be the primary traits developed in everyone.

However, reconstituting relationships in the public domain may well prove disruptive to contemporary notions of efficiency and effective functioning, which demand compliance from patients, children, nurses and family carers, with certain behaviour patterns and established routines, in order for organisations in turn to comply with pre-conceived definitions of function. In the case of hospitals, this may involve reducing waiting lists or increasing patient throughput without necessarily improving patient outcomes (McKee *et al.*, 1998).

On a broader note, as described in Chapter 3, the importance of addressing emotional and psychological needs as well as physical needs in promoting health, particularly in those suffering from long-term or chronic illness, is gaining recognition (Kaplun, 1992; Wass, 1994). Arguably, coercive environments that demand compliant behaviour with established routines are not conducive to meeting this type of need. As Baker's work illustrates, nurses attempting to establish non-coercive caring routines in hospital settings may well experience considerable difficulties and may themselves be construed as being inefficient and poor nurses by colleagues who are being judged and judging by very different criteria.

It follows that, although caring has been defined philosophically as a moral imperative and a universal human trait, the practices associated with caring on a daily basis have been marginalised and confined to the domestic arena. Here, family members gain the sustenance and nurturing that enables them to function effectively in the public domain. Where caring is required in public institutions, it is again ascribed to women, in particular low-paid women, who must conduct this work unobtrusively in order to ensure that it does not disrupt the public functions of the organisation.

The political invisibility of caring work

Finally, it is possible to highlight the relatively weak voice of both nurses and women in political arenas as a further parallel between nursing and women's work (Rafferty, 1992; Davies, 1995). Much of the literature provides a gender-based analysis of the invisibility of nursing in health care policy and attributes this to the predominance of women within the profession (Carpenter, 1993). The position of nursing within health care, it is argued, mirrors the position of women within society. A change in the status of nurses in health care will only come about if it is accompanied by a change in the status of women in society.

Robinson (1989) has addressed the issue of the marginalisation of nursing and women's work. She asks the question 'How can the activities and concerns of half a million waged nurses, and many more unpaid carers remain largely invisible in the policy arena?' (p. 151). Robinson suggests that part of the problem is located in the economics of caring. Unsurprisingly, given the definitions of caring as a universal human trait described earlier, the aptitude and inclination to care are in plentiful supply. This is encouraging if caring is found to be vital to human development. However, within an economy that places a high value on scarcity, the plentiful supply of something lowers its market value. Other essential prerequisites to health that are also in plentiful supply in advanced industrial countries, such as air and water, face the same problem and can be polluted because their plentiful supply means that they are both replaceable and expendable. Economics has yet to develop ways of valuing goods that are essential for health, such as caring, clean air and clean water, independently of the market economics of supply and demand (Capra, 1982).

Coupled with the economic problem, Robinson (1989) highlights the marginalisation of women's work as deriving from a failure in nursing and academic literature to analyse caring activities as a unified whole, regardless of whether the person undertaking the activity is receiving a wage for it. Robinson points out that, for some feminists, the development of waged carers such as nurses is argued to have led to the deskilling and devaluing of the intuitive and experientially learnt caring skills of women who stay at home.

Graham (1984) contrasts the importance of privacy and family (female) control over home-based caring activities with the moral obligations on families to use health services. As Graham notes, with some illnesses and some patients, securing medical help enhances a carer's status. Responsible parents attend antenatal classes, take their children to the dentist and child health clinic regularly and are quick to refer symptoms of concern to their doctor. In contrast, Graham reviews a range of studies suggesting that most parents are reluctant to involve outsiders in the process of care. Regardless of the difficulties experienced by families in caring for their sick or disabled members, the sanctity of the family must be maintained, even in the face of enormous personal cost; families feel that they must be seen to be coping. Consequently, Robinson (1989) points out that, when the caring work of women is transferred to the public domain and paid for by the health and social services, it is still regarded as being of such low skill and status that it does not require the investment of education and research.

Davies (1995) attributes the marginalisation of nursing in health care to the importance of gender in understanding how work comes to be defined and valued in public institutions. Davies describes how the notion of bureaucracy derives from a masculine logic that values impartiality, impersonality and hierarchy as key concepts in organising work. A similar logic, Davies argues, can be found to underpin the notion of 'profession', with its emphasis on expertise, detachment and autonomy. She goes on to argue that:

> Within a western cultural heritage, femininity – with its stress on dealing with dependency, acknowledging emotions and intimacy and nurturing others – comes to represent qualities that are feared and denied in masculinity, qualities that are best seen as to be contained and allocated to a different sphere, and at worst repressed and treated with contempt... Nursing, in other words, reminds us of the very vulnerabilities and dependencies that are edited out of masculinity. (Davies, 1995, p. 183)

Davies goes on to ask, 'Can nursing ever take its rightful place in policy debates about health care if this is what is at stake?' (Davies, 1995, p. 183).

Nursing, therefore, is caught in a double bind. In the public domain, it is still regarded as women's work and not worthy of investment. The key features of caring work stand in opposition to the main structures of bureaucracies and professions that characterise public institutions and in which status, power and rewards are located and distributed. When nurses do use their skills and knowledge to promote health, they are frequently viewed as agents of social control, usurping the primacy and privacy of the family and infringing individual liberty. This view is shared by feminists and by politicians of all political persuasions. Developing caring as a mainstream activity confronts more than the social taboos associated with physical care described by Lawler (1991): it also confronts the liberal principle of a human right to self-determination. Together, these present a formidable challenge to the intellectual development of nursing and the recognition of women's work as vital to the maintenance of health.

In recognition of the above debate, Robinson (1989) has called on waged nurses to reflect on the marginalisation of caring as women's work and to consider the case for increased mutual solidarity. Robinson suggests that this will require a recognition that caring is labour wherever it is carried out, and requires partnership across the sectors as well as appropriate rewards. Second, it requires a reconsideration of the gendered assumptions about the division of caring labour and a recognition of caring behaviours wherever they occur, regardless of the gender of the person performing them. Similarly, Davies (1995) has pointed out that men may also resist existing forms of 'the masculine vision' and in doing so may create 'a clash of masculinities' (p. 185) in which some men ally themselves with women in a bid for change.

Gender and status differentiation in health work

The marginalisation of nursing has also occurred within the management structures of health care institutions. Davies (1992) provides a cogent analysis of this literature. She points out that much of the literature on gender and nursing has been highly emotive and cast in pejorative language. The gender attributes applied to women and nurses include 'care commitment and self-sacrifice, on the one hand, and irrationality, indecisiveness and passivity on the other' (Davies, 1992, p. 236). Consequently, as Davies points out, several prominent analysts attribute the lack of progression made by female nurses in achieving senior management positions to inappropriate management behaviour portrayed by women and nurses. This in many ways sets up a circular argument in which inappropriate management behaviour on the part of female nurses is given as a reason for a lack of progression. At the same time, evidence of a lack of progression is used to label the behaviour traits of female nurses as inappropriate. As Davies points out, the lack of progression could give rise to the inappropriate behaviour rather than the other way round.

Davies, therefore, rejects this interpretation of female nurse management behaviour and instead introduces the concept of 'coping management'. Coping management is portrayed as an ineffective form of management (containing all the negative behaviour traits derived from empirical studies of nurse managers) practised by nurses, as a consequence of organisational neglect. Davies suggests that organisational neglect occurs because the practice-based (caring) concerns of nurses are not acknowledged and taken seriously by the organisation in which they work. This, Davies argues, gives rise to the dysfunctional behaviour frequently associated with nursing management. Davies's analysis suggests that this behaviour is not evidence of female inadequacy but instead a consequence of working in an organisation that devalues women and women's work.

This problem is not confined to nursing. Riska and Wegar (1993) illustrate the link between hierarchy, status and values in their analysis of the career paths of female doctors. They undertake a cross-cultural analysis of the careers of female doctors in Europe and America. Their findings highlight that, despite an increase in the proportion of female doctors (women now constituting 50 per cent of medical students in Britain), there has not been a corresponding increase in the proportion of women gaining high-status posts in management or hospital medicine. Instead, the career patterns of female doctors reveal a highly gendered division of labour. Most women doctors enter community medicine rather than hospital medicine, community medicine continuing to have a status subordinate to that of hospital medicine.

Riska and Wegar (1993) illustrate how the increase in the proportion of female doctors, without a corresponding increase in the total number of medical students, can be managed by the development of differential career paths in medicine. The increasing number of women doctors meets the increasing demand for community doctors. The decreasing proportion of male doctors retains control of the contracting hospital sector.

The above analysis recognises that work undertaken by females has been systematically devalued in a health service that places great status on the knowledge derived from the hard sciences and the subsequent technical interventions that this produces. From this perspective, the work of (both male and female) nurses, and of doctors who enter community medicine, appears to be menial, mundane and consequently not worthy of investment from scarce resources that could be used to pioneer new treatments.

The relatively weak position of nurses and women in the health service has been attributed to gendered organisational structures. These structures create barriers to progression for those with domestic commitments or those who place more value on the softer, less technical aspects of work. This provides a less judgemental analysis of the low status of female nurses than does a focus on the dysfunctional traits associated with female organisational behaviour (Davies, 1992). However, the actual behaviour portrayed by women as nurse managers is still deemed to be dysfunctional and, therefore, in some way inadequate. Certain behaviour traits portrayed predominantly by women are still labelled as dysfunctional, 'coping behaviours', while male attributes are still viewed as functional. Davies locates the problem for nurses in the disrespect shown by organisations to their work (labelled organisational neglect by Davies). This implies that if organisations could show respect for nursing, nurses would not adopt the dysfunctional behaviour traits currently portrayed as coping management but would instead be able to develop a more functional and constructive management style.

In contrast, Graham's work illustrates how coping is an integral aspect of caring. If this is the case, it may also be the case that the coping behaviours displayed by nurse managers and described by Davies (1992) are actually manifestations of caring behaviour rather than dysfunctional management traits. This provides an alternative explanation for the behaviour portrayed by female nurse managers, suggesting instead the continuation of caring as part of their learnt role. More theoretical and analytical work with regard to caring behaviours is required before a thorough understanding of the effectiveness of these behaviours in accomplishing caring within an organisational setting can be achieved.

Distinctions between nursing and family care

The previous section highlighted areas of overlap and commonality between nursing and family care. It is, however, clearly the case that they are not synonymous. Benner and Wrubel (1989) recognise that there are numerous differences, listing the distinctive differences as:

- *The role of the situation:* this acknowledges that while the situation within which nurse and patient meet might be familiar to the nurse, it is frequently an unfamiliar and unknown environment for the patient and the family. This is clearly not the case in family care. For the patient and family, the experience of health care is likely to be one that resonates with them for a long time and in which they search constantly for meaning. For the nurse, it could appear as mundane and routine.

- *The role of personal concern:* here it is suggested that family carers have a close emotional bond to the person being cared for, which is absent from most professional caring. Benner and Wrubel (1989) suggest that, in emergency situations or situations of new diagnosis, this closeness can interfere with judgement, giving rise to the need for strong professional care to manage the situation on behalf of the family. However, it is over time clearly the case that the particular understanding, shared family history and emotional commitment brought to the situation by the family carer will be an essential dimension of the caring process.

- *Temporality:* this refers to the different time frames within which professional carers and family carers interact with those for whom they care. Family carers have a long history of interpersonal relationships with the person being cared for. This is frequently intergenerational, the caring relationship being reciprocal between generations. Here, elderly parents are cared for in response to the care received by the carer as a child. As Bulmer (1987) notes, there is considerable concern not to undermine intergenerational reciprocity in caring through social policy provision that either leaves the burden too high for families to manage or completely takes over the responsibility, undermining the need for family care. This resonates with Benner and Wrubel's (1989) definition of caring as being about connecting with what matters. If we remove too many caring functions from families, we remove the core need for caring from society, creating increasing alienation and difficulty in identifying what is truly important from that which is merely topical. Similarly, James (1992) cautions against the formal extension of emotional labour into public health care structures, fearing that it will further expand medicine's territory, altering social relations in health care and creating further 'expertise' for sale abroad.

  For professional carers, caring is time-bound through shifts and time off duty. Benner and Wrubel (1989) see this time out as being essential for professional carers in order to renew their energy and allow time for reflection on their care-giving activities. As Benner and Wrubel (1989) note, family members are never 'off duty' in quite the same sense: although they may have time off from care-giving activities, they will have an ongoing relationship with the person being cared for, which is present with them wherever they go.

- *The role of embodied intelligence:* Benner and Wrubel (1989) suggest that nurses, through a repeated exposure to illness, build up an intuitive knowledge of and an increased sensitivity to the signs and symptoms of bodily functions. Newly diagnosed patients, on the other hand, have to acquaint themselves with the signs and symptoms of the illness as it manifests itself in their bodies, which may at first seem strange. In a later paper, Benner (1997) describes how nurses can work with patients to use the accumulated knowledge of nurses, patients and their family carers in order to refine and make better use of their embodied intelligence. Callery (1997), however, describes the difficulties experienced by mothers of sick children in conveying their concerns about their children to health care practitioners. He suggests that the problems arise from the difference between the knowledge base of the mother, which evolves in the private and intimate relationships of the family, and the knowledge of the professionals, which derives from the public domain of health care.

Other distinctions between nursing care and family care include: the time-limited relationship of the nurse as against the ongoing relationship of the family carer; the relatively public role of the nurse compared with the essentially private role of the family carer; the scope of professional practice (UKCC, 1992) in the UK provides the public interpretation of the role of the nurse, and the absence of such a document for family care; and the right for the nurse to have time 'off duty', no similar right existing for family carers.

Finally, Kitson (1987), in a comparative analysis of lay caring and professional (nursing) caring, concludes that '[Lay] Caring and nursing seem to be inextricably bound together in terms of the concepts shared and activities performed' (Kitson, 1987, p. 164). The shared concepts and attributes identified by Kitson include commitment, knowledge and skills, and respect for persons. She suggests that what differentiates lay care from professional care is the fact that professional care provides those aspects of care which the lay carer (or person) cannot provide because of a lack of commitment, resources, knowledge or skill. It would seem that nursing cannot escape the dilemma of intrusion into lay family care if it is to fulfil its potential. The moral and ethical framework in which it takes this remit forward is clearly crucial to the effectiveness of this endeavour.

Future directions for nursing care

In response to the problems of marginalisation and lack of professional identity found in nursing, Boeije *et al.* (1997) undertook an analysis of future possible scenarios for nursing in the Netherlands. In undertaking the analysis, they distinguished between ambiguous and unambiguous forces driving nursing forward. Unambiguous forces were identified as demographic and epidemiological trends such as those portrayed in Chapter 3. These trends were relatively predictable and stable. The ambiguous forces identified in the study as influencing the future demand for nursing care were:

- patient emancipation, arising from an increasing demand on the part of patients to be given more say in how their lives were run;

- the role of informal carers in contributing to care.

The critical uncertainties confronting the supply of nurses were:

- task interpretation and task execution by nurses and home carers, this relates to the interpretation of the role and function of nurses by patients and by other professionals who may be changing the boundaries of the service they offer;

- the restructuring and modernisation of nursing and home care financing, which relates to the sources and level of funding made available, collectively and privately, for nursing and home care.

Boeije *et al.* (1997) identified two types of professional nursing. First is that carried out by the diagnosis-orientated nurse, whose work is driven by functional indicators of effectiveness within research-tested interventions. This approach to nursing sets boundaries on what constitutes nursing work and on the relationship between nurses and other health care professionals. Second is the needs-orientated approach to nursing, the nurse's work addressing the meaning of an illness for the person concerned. Here, the primary concern is to increase the well-being of the person. The needs-orientated approach more closely incorporates the key concerns with caring discussed above.

Boeije *et al.* (1997) suggest that centrally managed provision, as in the NHS, is usually based on some form of needs assessment to which service provision is matched. This will facilitate the work of diagnosis-orientated nurses, who will be able to identify the contribution that they can make to meet the needs of specific diagnostic groups. In contrast, centrally managed provision based on a catchment area scenario, such as that being developed under HAZs in the UK, should facilitate the work of needs-orientated nurses. These nurses work in partnership with patients and local populations to identify meaning and provide services designed to improve the quality of life across the whole population.

The significance of Boeije *et al.*'s work is that it lifts the debate on the future of nursing from a position of preoccupation with status and subordination, to one that locates the significance of nursing work in the wider debates about the future direction of health care funding and provision. This enables nurses to identify options and influence the direction of provision. In so doing, they of necessity influence their own futures. The next section extends the work of Boeije *et al.* and reviews the potential contribution of nursing to meeting the major health needs of the population identified in Chapter 3.

Needs analysis and the role of carers

The work of Boeije *et al.* (1997) highlights the critical role of care work as a focus for policy. The way in which nurses develop their role, allocate their time and distribute nursing resources will have a major impact on future demands for caring services. This is illustrated in the social policy literature that consistently highlights the adverse impact of care work on opportunities for informal carers to exercise individual autonomy. Baldwin and Twigg (1991, p. 124), in a review of the research on informal care, summarise the findings as follows:

- that the care of non-spousal dependent people falls primarily to women;
- that it is unshared to a significant extent by relatives, statutory or voluntary agencies;
- that it creates burdens and material costs which are a source of significant inequalities between men and women;
- that many women nevertheless accept the role of informal carer and, indeed, derive satisfaction from doing so;
- that the reasons for this state of affairs are deeply bound up with the construction of female and male identity, and possibly also with culturally defined rules about gender appropriate behaviours.

It is possible that nursing, by augmenting family care, is instrumental in sustaining and maintaining informal carers in the community. What evidence there is suggests that this burden will fall disproportionately on the female members of the family. The issue is complicated by the fact that, in their concern for their family, women will often willingly accept the additional care burden and will seek satisfaction in their ability to provide excellent care to family members.

From the perspective of health economists, such a situation appears to be wholly acceptable: women as competent adults faced with a dependent family member choose to spend their time seeking the satisfaction that can be derived from looking after that family member effectively. The inequality arises from the fact that, in choosing to do this, women are of necessity forgoing the opportunity to pursue other life goals or, within our current system of economic distribution, to establish economic independence, which, it could be argued, is a foundation for their autonomy as adults. The link between autonomy, independence, self-determination and health described in Chapter 2 suggests that if women take on the role of carers, they are subject to social and material inequalities that are simultaneously recognised as giving rise to ill-health.

In recognition of this, Finch (1984) recommends the physical removal of people who cannot manage without extensive support into institutional care. This, she suggests, is the only way in which women can be freed from the moral coercion to care and be enabled to achieve the state of independence and autonomy philosophically defined by many (Seedhouse, 1986; Doyal and Gough, 1991) as the hallmark of adult status and, simultaneously, of health. The solution advocated by Finch, while extreme, is illuminating in that it forces a confrontation of the assumptions upon which community care policies operate and in which nurses may become the unwitting vehicles for the coercion of family members, in reality women, to take on the role of carer. In so doing, nurses would be instrumental in perpetuating structural inequalities in society.

In reviewing the arguments put forward by Finch (1984), Baldwin and Twigg (1991) have tried to assert a middle path. They argue for the recognition of a collective responsibility for people unable to survive independently. This can be delegated but not to the extent that those who take on the task of discharging this collective responsibility are prevented from 'leading relatively ordinary lives' (Baldwin and Twigg, 1991, p. 132). Additionally, Baldwin and Twigg suggest that, as carers are discharging a collective responsibility, they have a right to support and compensation from the collective on whose behalf they are discharging this responsibility.

The definition of 'relatively ordinary lives' indicates the importance of the recognition of relative need as a basis for policy (Bradshaw, 1972). The recognition of collective responsibility, however, augments this definition. It suggests that the definition of carer need should not just be based on comparison with other carers. This could lead to a situation in which the needs of a given carer would be compared with the needs of other carers, all of whom were leading the lives of relatively ordinary carers. Consequently, they would all be subject to the same level of moral coercion and economic inequality that characterises the lives of all carers. Instead, the importance of collective responsibility indicates that needs analysis should be based on a theoretical foundation. One such theoretical foundation is provided by Seedhouse (1986) who, in his formulation of a theoretical foundation for health, attempts to identify the basic needs required by all individuals, which would include carers, to achieve health.

In contrast, however, Benner and Wrubel (1989) suggest that it is not care work itself that is damaging, but the economic inequality associated with low wages or no wages at all that tends to accompany it. Benner and Wrubel would dispute definitions of health based on the realisation of autonomy and independence as essentially male-orientated definitions of health. In defining care as work that matters to the people performing it, in particular family carers, but also nurses and other care workers, Benner and Wrubel highlight the intrinsic satisfaction to be derived from care work, which ultimately connects the work with thinking and with feelings. Consequently, Benner and Wrubel suggest that the concepts of autonomy and independence that promote individual satisfaction separate people from the things they care about most, and this can give rise to feelings of anomie and alienation.

For Benner and Wrubel, the universal definition of caring as a human moral imperative does not result in caring activities being experienced as worthy burdens, but instead provides an important source of human satisfaction and fulfilment. Undertaking care work is, therefore, not something to be avoided as an adult because it reduces life opportunities but something to be embraced for the satisfactions it brings.

Summary

Chapter 3 indicated that the biggest challenge facing health service planners at the start of the 21st century is not the ageing of the population in itself, but the escalating cost of medical technology and the inappropriate use of much of this technology. The solution to this problem was seen to reside in the development of primary health care, in which secondary (hospital) care becomes increasingly specialist, accessed only by those for whom there is sound clinical evidence that they can benefit from such technology. Chapter 3 also indicated that, as the population ages, the incidence of chronic disease rises, impacting on the demand for technology. If secondary care is to fulfil its function in clinical effectiveness, the integration of technology into the everyday lives of patients must be successfully achieved. This means that patients and their families must be given the support needed to accept and learn how to live fulfilling lives within the limitations imposed by illness and dependency. A failure in any part of this is likely to rebound the patient back into secondary care.

This chapter has demonstrated that the major challenges facing nursing at the start of the 21st century are the emancipation of patients and their families, and the interpretation placed on the role of the nurse in the context of care. There appears, however, to be something of a contradiction in the literature on caring and caring relationships. It is now well documented that adult physical and mental health derives in part from the quality of the caring relationship experienced as a child (Blaxter, 1981; Graham, 1984; Reder and Lucey, 1995). However, social policy has been reluctant to breach the public/private divide and still holds the family as being sacrosanct, as providing a retreat from the pressures of public life and therefore to be safeguarded from intrusion by public agencies (Froland, 1980; Bulmer, 1987). Similarly, in health and social care practice, largely unqualified staff (James, 1992) carry out much of the work associated with caring.

The removal of caring from the public sphere adopts a universal definition of caring based on a combination of common sense and humanity. It assumes that caring is an innate aspect of humanity, that both parties to the caring relationship are reasonable, well-adjusted people and that both professional and family carers always work in the best interest of those for whom they care regardless of circumstances.

The removal of caring from the public sphere has the added advantage of rendering 'safe' the potentially controversial outcomes of professionalising the caring process. However, the removal of caring from the public sphere also contradicts the growing body of evidence indicating that the quality of relationships between patients and professional carers, and also between parents and children, can work either to promote or to detract from health outcomes (Blaxter, 1981; Kelly and May, 1982; Graham, 1984; Thorne and Robinson, 1989; Reder and Lucey, 1995). If the health and social services are to remain significant in addressing some of the more fundamental problems facing health maintenance and promotion, they cannot afford to ignore this growing body of evidence.

Whitbeck (1984), Kitson (1987) and Robinson (1989) have all highlighted the similarities between family care and nursing care, and have sought to identify the competencies associated with effective caring relationships, wherever they are located and regardless of who carries them out. In contrast, the social policy literature has been characterised by a recognition of the contradictions and discontinuities that exist between the informal relationships that characterise family and community care, and the formal relationships deriving from professional and public services. Concern has been expressed about usurping family caring roles by adopting an overinterventionist stance (Bulmer, 1987; Coyne, 1995). However, Lipsky (1991) has recognised that, in providing responsive services sensitive to individual circumstances, some degree of worker discretion and intervention is necessary and tolerated by public agencies. The literature on caring has evolved within this paradox. A concern about usurping family caring roles means that professional caring relationships have been seen as being based on common sense and humanity, which denies the complexity of achieving these relationships in practice. This has rendered nursing and caring work invisible in health and social care institutions (Robinson, 1989; Davies, 1992).

The policy shift to primary care means an inevitable increase in demand for informal family care. As this chapter demonstrates, nurses, in practice and in theory, act at the interface between formal and informal care. How they interpret their role, allocate nursing resources and influence the allocation of social care resources may fundamentally affect the extent to which both patients and informal family carers are enabled to live 'relatively ordinary lives'. In attempting to understand the processes by which the interweaving of formal and informal care can be successfully accomplished, the experiences of nurses, other paid carers and women may be particularly revealing. It follows, therefore, that if nurses' and carers' voices continue to be subordinate in the planning of provision, as depicted by Robinson (1989), Davies (1995) and Smith and Agard (1997), the chances of primary health care policies succeeding are severely compromised. The next chapter looks at how nurses and carers work together to manage care at the interface between formal and informal care and to resolve problems arising from the cultural ethos and structural boundaries that currently characterises provision.

Chapter 5

Accomplishing Caring as Labour

The previous chapter indicated how 'care as labour' is primarily located in the informal and privatised structures associated with family provision. This care is supplemented by formal care provided by nurses and other care workers in the public domain. 'Care as labour' work in the public domain shares many, although by no means all, of the characteristics of care carried out privately by family members.

Bulmer (1987) has noted the increasing attention being paid to informal care in public policy. This, he suggests, is derived from the need to make statutory and non-statutory services complementary to one another, with the particular aim of postponing the need for residential or institutional care for as long as possible. As Bulmer emphasises, the success of this approach depends largely on the ability to mobilise various forms of family or informal care.

This chapter reviews some of the ways in which nurses organise themselves to accomplish 'care as labour'. It starts with a description of nursing as a responsive activity, sensitive not only to the biopsychosocial needs of the patient, but also to the network of complex organisational structures within which health and social care are delivered. Three models of care provision derived from the work of Kitson (1993) are presented and analysed, and the decision-making processes embedded in 'care as labour' are discussed. The chapter concludes with a discussion of the types of behaviour that accomplish 'care as labour' and the problems of accommodating these types of behaviour within mainstream, hierarchical organisational structures.

Nursing: a responsive activity

The contribution of nursing care to hospital patients is frequently distinguished by the fact that nurses (collectively rather than individually) are with the patients 24 hours a day every day of the year. Many nurses extol the virtues of this level of provision and claim a greater knowledge and understanding of the patient, as well as a greater opportunity to educate the patient, because of this sustained contact (Kuhse, 1997).

From this perspective, the virtue of nursing seems to reside in the context of 'being with the patient' (McKee, 1991; Radwin, 1996). Indeed, the idea of 'being with' patients as a basis for practice has been given increased credibility by a number of nurse theorists, using predominantly phenomenological perspectives (Benner and Wrubel, 1989; Morse *et al.*, 1991; Brykczynska, 1997). A similar case is made in midwifery (Davies, 1995).

The concept of 'being with' the patient as a legitimate activity and basis for practice has to be set against the more instrumental, therapeutic and episodic interventions associated with medicine and the professions allied to medicine. In fact, one of the major problems confronting the development of a research base to nursing practice is the identification of discrete therapeutic nursing interventions that can be evaluated (Bond and Thomas, 1991; Kitson, 1997).

This is not to say that nurses do not intervene in patient care: they clearly do. However, the basis for the intervention is rarely derived solely from nursing knowledge. Almost every nursing activity, from the administration of drugs to feeding, positioning or communicating with patients, has a knowledge base that is the specialist province of some other health care professional. It is possible to argue that nurses, in their daily care of patients, act inevitably as surrogates for most other health care professionals, but rarely as professionals in their own right.

If nurses in their daily care activities are acting as surrogates for other health care professionals, it follows that they are not the ones who prescribe or initiate treatment, their role instead being restricted to one of implementation. This could be in relation to drug therapy, physiotherapy, speech therapy, counselling or occupational therapy. Nurses are, therefore, responding to the treatment needs prescribed by other health care professionals. In this way, they are not in control of their knowledge base or their workload; this remains the province of those outside nursing practice.

In this context, the 24-hour provision of care becomes the distinguishing feature of nursing on which the value of nursing can be assessed. In order to understand nursing, therefore, it is necessary to understand the claim that nurses are the providers of 24-hour care for patients. This is the key to both the knowledge base of nursing and the organisation and structure of nursing provision.

Nurses as individuals clearly cannot give 24-hour care. This requires some form of labour substitution. The nature and organisation of the labour substitution in nursing has been the subject of a large body of research (discussed in Chapters 7 and 8) and, as the previous chapter illustrates, is structured into the delivery of 'care as labour' regardless of who is providing this care. It is important, however, also to understand how 24-hour provision affects the knowledge base in nursing. Recognising that nurses, as individuals, cannot provide 24-hour care has led one MSc student to describe the nature of nursing work as 'the responsibility for the 24-hour life space of the patient' (Croom, 1996, p. 2).

This phrase makes an important theoretical contribution to understanding the nature of nursing work. It suggests that, in managing the 24-hour provision of care, nursing is responsible for integrating the world of the patient with that of the service. Nursing creates the web within which other professions practise. Nurses act at the interface between the areas of physical, psychological, emotional and social disorder created for the patient and their relatives/informal carers by the onset or progression of the illness, and the ordered, regulated, labelled and controlled environments demanded by bureaucracies in order to schedule episodic therapeutic interventions (for example, investigations, surgery, drug therapy, psychology, physiotherapy and occupational therapy).

From this perspective, nurses are, in fact, the key to efficiency within hospitals. Poor nursing will give rise to an inefficient organisation. Equally, however, organisations are the key to efficiency in nursing. Non-responsive, highly bureaucratised organisations, which do not adapt easily to the individual needs of patients, are likely to be difficult environments for nurses to work in (James, 1994).

While this may be more obvious in hospital nursing, it is also true in community nursing. Here, there is a need to enable patients and family carers to live 'relatively ordinary lives', as depicted by Baldwin and Twigg (1991) and discussed in the previous chapter. Family carers require support to make decisions and to access the resources required to meet their own personal needs, as well as the needs of the dependent relative. This may require nurses to understand and work with the dynamic power relations found within the family and to enable carers to work through feelings of moral coercion to care and guilt if they do not, which are structured into the gendered role of many women (Finch, 1984; Graham, 1984). Such work may be crucial if carers are to sustain their role over the long term and not themselves succumb to illness or economic inequality, which will create further problems at a later stage in their life.

All of this work fits in with and derives from the concept of the management of the 24-hour life space of the patient. This work is highly complex as it appears on the surface to invade the private decisions of carers, as competent adults, to decide how they live their lives and how they care for their families. There is some evidence that community nurses can and do undertake this work (Gould, 1996; ENB, 1999). There is also evidence that families looking after a sick person at home can sometimes be overwhelmed by the number of specialists who call round. Nurses have a key role to play in co-ordinating inputs to ensure that families are supported but also have some space for themselves (ENB, 1999).

Planning for uncertainty

Planners tend to work with statistics that highlight stability in patterns over time, so their information sources are very different from those of nurses. While the general incidence of a given disease may be well known, nurses confront the unfortunate individual so soon to become a health service statistic.

For this individual, the illness or accident may well be a complete surprise, causing considerable shock for themselves and their family, employer, colleagues and friends. In the person's personal life, this was not a predictable and planned-for event. Consequently, all sorts of aspects of life are thrown into complete disorder. This disorder may have serious implications for people other than the patient. Dependants, including children, elderly relatives, neighbours, dogs, cats and budgies, are at varying degrees of short- or long-term risk, while the patient, caught up in the drama of health care, is temporarily powerless to respond. Good nursing enables a response, thus locating the onset of illness or accident in the wider web of the patient's life and concerns. This type of nursing action alleviates anxiety for the patient (Newman, 1984) and allows the patient to focus on and be receptive to the health care interventions being provided by the health service.

From the patient's perspective, illness is a precarious experience, its onset, progression and outcome usually being unexpected, unstable and unknown. The treatments, however, are scheduled to meet bureaucratic imperatives. They are prescribed to conform to routine practices, which maximise the effective use of health service resources (theatres, X-rays, laboratories, screening and wound dressings). In the community, scheduling visits to specialists or enabling families to access health care services requires a fit between the schedules of professionals and the schedules of and demands being made on the family. The uncertainty for the organisation arising from the precarious nature of illness is, as far as possible, replaced by an ordered regimen, providing the illusion of certainty. Triage may be an example of this (Read, 1994).

Alternatively, the patient might be accessing health service resources because of the progression of an existing medical condition. Again, the progression can be unexpected and the outcome unknown. The patient's life is, similarly, temporarily disordered by this development. However, the patient does have a previous experience of the illness and the effects of previous treatments on the illness and him or herself. A denial, by the health care providers, of this experience can create considerable anxiety for patients, reducing their effectiveness as patients (Thorne, 1993; Lyons *et al.*, 1995).

For health service planners, certainty is captured in health service statistics that provide fairly stable and reliable data on the expected incidence of disease by diagnosis, age, gender and geographical location (see Chapter 3). This should, in theory, enable the provision of services to be planned to match the expected demand. In reality, however, service providers frequently experience a mismatch between planned provision and demand, giving rise to long waiting times and considerable short-term pressure on resources (Clarke, 1996).

Planners and providers, therefore, despite reliable and fairly stable data, also require systems that enable them to *cope* with the fluctuations in demand that arise on a daily basis, derived from the uncertainty experienced at an individual level at the onset or progression of illness. Attempts to manage the uncertainty surrounding the onset or progression of illness without understanding the nature of the uncertainty often result in setting up systems that merely divert the uncertainty to another department but do not resolve it. Examples of this include the setting up of overnight admission wards attached to accident and emergency (A&E) departments. These wards resolve the disruption to the ordinary wards at night but further fragment the care received by the patient, simultaneously failing to tackle the uncertainty surrounding the demand for emergency admission to hospitals at night.

To summarise, therefore, it is possible to suggest that nursing mediates between the uncertainty experienced by the patient and the family in accessing health care, and the organisational demand to manage the patient's progress within and through the system in a routine and predictable way. Nursing thus ensures that patients are both referred for and prepared for treatment and are available in the right place, in the right condition (physical, social, psychological and emotional) at the right time.

In order to do this, nurses transmit information from the patient to the organisation to ensure that the organisation can provide appropriate services for the patient, for example an immobile patient who requires a wheelchair, or vegetarian who needs a vegetarian diet. Nurses also transmit information from the service to the patient ensuring that the patient knows and understands the various investigations and treatments planned for them, for example the need to fast for four hours prior to a given investigation, or that it is normal to feel some pain after a given procedure.

At the same time, nurses respond to the specific needs of patients and carers as they arise during the course of their illness. As well as ensuring compliance with treatment programmes prescribed by other health care professionals, nurses also attend to the comfort and privacy of the patient. Consequently, nurses manage aspects of daily bodily functioning such as: access to the toilet as required; access to an adequate nutritional and fluid intake; the management of pain control; and responding to the social and emotional needs and anxieties of patients as they arise during the course of care. Any or all of these can be temporarily disrupted by the illness, investigations or prescribed treatment.

Learning how to interweave formal and informal care through nursing practice

The above description of nursing care suggests that it practises at the focal point between formal and informal care. Nursing, therefore, operates at the interface between creating dependence and independence; between partnerships based on professional expertise and definitions of need, and partnerships based on patient expertise and definitions of need; between a 'nanny state' of interference and a 'self-reliant' state that can give rise to neglect. It does this initially and primarily within a legislative context in which free access to medical treatment and technology is enshrined within government policy legislation, but no similar free access to care as labour is guaranteed or expected.

At a fundamental level nursing, therefore, derives legitimacy to practise from the needs for 'care as labour' that arise out of medically directed interventions (Kuhse, 1997). Through this legitimacy, however, nursing is able to develop a body of theoretical and practical expertise about 'care as labour' that has relevance to situations beyond the narrow confines of medical interventions. This expertise could inform wider social policy concerns that arise at the interface between the provision of formal and informal care.

The complexity of state interference in personal relationships is explored by Twigg (1989), who identifies three major contradictions that she suggests characterise the relationship between informal carers and formal service provision.

The first is the tension between prevention and substitution; here, the concern is that early intervention designed to support carers and strengthen their involvement in caring for their families will in fact have the reverse effect and substitute for informal care, encouraging people to do less for their dependants.

The second contradiction reflects the concerns of Finch (1984) and Baldwin and Twigg (1991) described in the previous chapter. Here, conflicts of interest are recognised between the dependant's need for care and the carer's independence and right to function as an autonomous adult. However, concentrating on carer stress without recognising that people can and do choose to continue to do things that cause them considerable distress, undermines the importance of caring as a focal human activity in favour of the value of autonomy.

The third contradiction relates to targeting. In this area, debates ensue about whether resources should be targeted at those who are expressing difficulties with caring, even if the demands are light, or those who on objective assessment fit criteria that indicate a high level of carer burden. As Twigg points out, there is evidence suggesting that male carers abandon care giving at lower levels of both objective burden and subjectively expressed stress. If this is the case, policies using either of these measures are likely to reinforce gender biases in care giving.

Each of the contradictions identified by Twigg occurs at the interface between informal care and formal provision. While clearly a matter for policy analysts, these dilemmas are in practice resolved every day through the allocation of nursing resources and the way in which nursing is practised within the context of these dilemmas. As Boeije *et al.* (1997) found, how and in what circumstances nursing care is provided and the ways in which it is implemented determine the ethical resolution of these central policy questions. This analysis suggests that the ethical resolution of caring problems is embedded in the fabric of nursing behaviours. It is possible to suggest that this domain not only presents nursing with the most formidable challenge, but also provides the focus for considerable intellectual endeavour from which new understandings about how to cross this 'frontier' (Abrams, 1980) may emerge.

Decision making in nursing care

The above discussion of nursing illustrates how nurses work at the interface between the patients' experience of illness and the disruptive and anxiety-provoking nature of this experience, and the integration of this potentially volatile situation into the smooth regimes and eligibility criteria demanded by rational-legal organisational structures. In this context, caring for patients is about finding out what matters to them, finding out what matters to the organisation and negotiating between the two domains. The outcome of these negotiations reflects organisational protocols and procedures, adapted to individual need, which in turn resolve the theoretical tensions in policy described by Twigg (1989) above.

This aspect of nursing can be discerned in the work of Kitson (1993), who has developed a conceptual framework for caring derived from theoretical progression in nursing scholarship. This framework identifies three forms of caring that are found in nursing: caring-as-duty, caring-as-therapeutic-relationship, and caring-as-ethical-position.

Caring-as-duty derived, according to Kitson (1993), from the gendered role of women in which the caring role of the woman (that is, the nurse) was seen to have high moral and religious overtones. Structures were created in which devotion, dedication, vocation, obedience and submissiveness became the hallmarks of a good nurse and a good woman. The caring-as-duty paradigm can still be detected in some areas of nursing and, as the next chapter reveals, is in danger of being reinvented in a new occupation of generic worker as nurses assert a knowledge-based approach to practice.

According to Kitson, caring-as-duty is characterised by a task-orientated approach to care, which is carried out unthinkingly by an obedient nurse. This approach was also characterised by rapid turnover, a high wastage rate and poor-quality care. Menzies (1960), in a seminal study into the organisation of nursing care, found that the discontinuity and fragmentation that characterised provision distanced nurses from patients, enabling nurses to avoid engaging with patient experiences. On the surface, this created efficiency, but it left nurses in denial of their feelings, with unresolved anxieties arising from their work to which they could not give expression. Consequently, nurses became distressed and disillusioned, while patients felt isolated and neglected.

If we relate caring-as-duty back to the definitions of health given in Chapter 2, it is possible that, at its best, caring-as-duty could give rise to some functional outcomes for patients in that they might be kept clean, tidy and well nourished. It could, however, lead to a neglected environment, in which a failure to care for the feelings and emotions of nurses was accompanied by a failure to care for the patients (Davies, 1992; Tschudin, 1997).

Caring-as-therapeutic-relationship, according to Kitson, arose out of the work of nurse theorists from the 1960s onwards, particularly in the USA (Mayeroff, 1972; Rogers, 1980). For these writers, the process of caring was viewed as inherently therapeutic. Features of caring such as empathy, sympathy, trust, hope, love, honesty and respect were analysed and incorporated into theories to inform nursing practice. Feelings were allowed to surface in nursing, and nurses were encouraged to link self with other and to encourage mutual disclosure and sharing.

Many of the nursing theories and models developed at this time were derived in part from psychology and in part from pyschodynamic theory. Nursing, however, also involves physical contact, which rarely forms a component of psychotherapeutic encounters. Moreover, as this chapter argues, a distinguishing feature of nursing is a theoretical understanding, structuring and integration of the 24-hour care needs of patients. This involves the need both to anticipate and respond to situations, and to deal with emotions as they arise in and through daily activities such as eating, sleeping, dressing, socialising and leisure.

This is quite different from the episodic and quasi-anonymous interventions thought to be appropriate for psychotherapy to accomplish its task (Budd, 1994). As Kitson notes, the extent to which therapeutic relationships based on the principles of psychotherapy can be effectively managed in the context of the intimate and continuous caring work carried out by nurses has not been fully explored.

Nursing-as-therapeutic-relationship reflects concerns about growth in understanding by both parties. In practice, it links back to the concepts of health associated with developmental philosophies, empowerment philosophies and concepts of health as well-being described in Chapter 2.

Caring-as-ethical-position derived, according to Kitson, from the work of Watson (1985) and Benner and Wrubel (1989). Here, as in care-as-duty, morality and ethics feature strongly. This time, however, nurses are seen as autonomous practitioners who use their understanding of the dynamics of the patient situation to make good decisions or correct judgements. Here, the nurse undertakes the full range of tending activities and, through these, shares with the patient, and bears witness to, the experiences of the illness. According to Benner and Wrubel (1989), nursing becomes a means by which patients can maintain their human identity and integrity in the face of illness. The nurse searches for and identifies how patients live their lives, in order to help them to identify how they can live with their illness and ultimately their death.

If we return to the definitions of health given in Chapter 2, it is clear that this position could give rise to the realisation of growth and development as the nurse and patient explore the different dimensions of the illness. It could also reinforce the patient's ability to cope with the illness, transferring strategies used to cope with everyday life into the repertoire of strategies used to cope with the illness. As Kitson notes, there are many overlaps and similarities between care-as-therapeutic-relationship and care-as-ethical-position. In the therapeutic position, a number of rules and principles of psychotherapeutic practice are used to govern decision making; in the ethical paradigm, each rule has to be considered on its merits in the context of the evolving relationship and mutual realisation of the situation.

The different dimensions of the three paradigms described by Kitson are illustrated in the following vignettes of nursing practice. These are introduced to illustrate how formal and informal care converge in nursing and give rise to an holistic (for a discussion of how holism is being used here, see Chapter 2) understanding of the situation at the point of problem solving.

The first vignette highlights the complexities that nurses face when formal and informal care decisions converge. In this, the nurses were not instrumental in the decision to admit the patient, but they clearly had to manage the consequences of this decision. They were powerless to influence the future for this patient so could not negotiate a compromise with her. As a consequence, all were prisoners of the decisions of absent and authoritative parties. This had direct implications for the standard of care that the nurses were able to provide to this patient and to other patients on the ward, which fell below what the nurses considered acceptable. The self-esteem of all of those involved was, therefore, undermined by these decisions. By excluding the nurses and the patient

Vignette

The nurses who removed the Zimmer frame

This case was observed while collecting data for the author's PhD thesis (Procter, 1989b). An elderly patient had recently been admitted to a long-stay care of the elderly ward. The ward was of the traditional Nightingale design, with 30 beds. The incident was observed during the course of an evening shift. There were three nurses on duty: a state enrolled nurse and two auxiliaries. The patient was unhappy about her admission to the ward and repeatedly told the nurses that she wanted to go home. She lived by herself in an isolated rural setting some distance from her family. It was the middle of winter and very cold. Her family did not think that she could manage alone at home and were instrumental in getting her admitted to the ward.

After a few hours of repeatedly explaining her desire to go home, to which the nurses listened sympathetically, the elderly lady walked, using her Zimmer frame, to the ward doors in an attempt to leave. The ward exited onto the perimeter road of the hospital. The nurses caught the patient at the second set of doors, but she refused to return to her bedside. The nurses cajoled, encouraged and physically returned her to her bed. The patient immediately repeated the exercise. One nurse guarded the ward doors, the other nurse rang the patient's relatives, described what was happening and asked them to talk to the patient, which they did to no avail. The situation continued, occupying two and sometimes all three nurses for the next hour. Other patients were being neglected. In the end, the nurses reluctantly removed the Zimmer frame. The patient protested long and loudly about this. The nurses were busy catching up with the neglected needs of all the other patients.

After a while, the patient needed to go to the toilet, but she was unable to get there without her Zimmer frame, nor could she attract the attention of a nurse; she eventually urinated on the floor. The nurses expressed their exasperation at her behaviour as they cleaned her up and mopped the floor. The patient looked humiliated. As the nurses were going off duty, the patient offered them some chocolate as a token of reconciliation. The nurses refused it.

from the decision-making process, the nurses were forced to work within the care-as-duty paradigm, with its emphasis on tasks and blind obedience to the decisions of others. The refusal to accept the chocolate is reflective of Menzies' description of fragmented care, in which nurses distance themselves from the object of their care; in this case, they did not want to share the patient's humiliation, which was a product of the situation in which she found herself.

This vignette also illustrates the knowledge that those who 'bear witness' to the situation by their engagement in caring gain about the situation. This understanding provides a legitimate alternative source of information, which is fundamental to a successful resolution of caring problems. This point is made by Kuhse (1997), who argues that it is precisely the different knowledge gained through continuous caring, rather than episodic interventions, that gives nursing its unique perspective on ethical decisions.

According to Benner and Wrubel (1989), nursing is characterised by sharing the illness experience with the patient in order to understand how to enable the patient to live successfully through this experience. However, as the above vignette illustrates, nurses can only accomplish this if they are active participants in the decision-making process. This means that nurses must be enabled to influence the outcome of the decision for patients and to help both patients and families to address the underlying problems, of which the behaviour of the patient in Vignette 1 was merely a symptom. To deny carers (including nurses) any involvement in decision making while expecting them to 'bear witness' to the care creates a spoilt identity for nurses in which their self-esteem can only be preserved at the patient's expense.

Tschudin (1997) describes how, when the emotional needs of nurses for self-respect and self-esteem are not met, there then arises in nurses the need to control and rule so as not to be at the mercy of someone or something else. In such circumstances, Tschudin suggests, the shadow of the symbol of nursing surfaces, in which nurses split themselves off from the supporting aspects of their role and blindly follow the demands of 'the system'. The above discussion of the role of nursing at the interface between the uncertainty of the patient's situation and the regulation demanded by bureaucracies illustrates the problems that will be created for patients if nurses blindly follow 'the system'. Nurses are then subject to the negative influences of following 'the system', as illustrated in Vignette 1 above, which in turn creates ill-health in themselves and their patients.

Vignette 2 highlights the adaptations to normal care and treatment routines that might have to be made to accommodate family circumstances. Nurses responsible for managing this type of care need sufficient clinical knowledge to make an informed decision about these

---

Vignette 2

Enabling blind parents to care for a sick child at home

Gould (1996), a community children's nurse, describes the home care management of a two-and-a-half-year-old child suffering from cancer. Both parents were blind and reliant upon guide dogs, and there was also an older child in the family to be looked after. Following an unplanned discharge, the parents were taught how to manage each aspect of their child's care. Normal routine family care, such as bathing, was complicated by the presence of a central line and urinary catheter, which were taped with white tape as the child's mother was able to see white. The child's father was encouraged to cut his child's hair, as he had always done, even though the scissors at times came very close to the central line. The parents were taught how to check the position of the central line and catheter, and to check that they had not become dislodged. They were also taught what to do should this occur. It is usually recommended that disposable gloves be worn when emptying the catheter bag of a patient receiving cytotoxic therapy, but in this case the parents' reliance on touch to complete procedures prevented the use of gloves. Finally, it was necessary to bring in a social services carer to help with some aspects of family care. In doing this, it was important that both the carer and the parents understood their role and worked out together the responsibilities of the social services carer.

---

adaptations and to know what can and cannot be changed in the light of family circumstances. They also have to make ethical decisions about the degree of responsibility that they can entrust to the parents described in this vignette, in order to enable the parents to continue in their parenting role without engendering dependency or leaving the parents vulnerable to a failure to cope. In Vignette 2, the nurse was able to work in partnership with the parents and to exercise considerable professional judgement within the context of this partnership. The shadow of nursing found in Vignette 1 is absent.

Vignettes 1 and 2 also illustrate how the biopsychosocial and affective or emotional dimensions of an individual or family situation manifest in the everyday practice of nursing, without nurses having to undertake any huge conceptual leaps from one paradigm to another. In their practice nurses also 'bear witness' to the impact, on patients, of current configurations of service provision, which may exacerbate or ameliorate the resolution of a caring problem. All of these dimensions are simply there. Care-as-labour performed as part of nursing, therefore, offers the potential to explore the integration of 'formal' and 'informal' care through an analysis of nurses' everyday encounters with

---

Vignette 3

All for the want of an epi-syringe

This vignette describes the care received by a family with a child with pituitary gland deficiency. The mother reported the incident during an interview for a research project (ENB, 1999). Following the diagnosis, the family was referred to the local community children's nursing service to commence daily hormone injections. The nurses visited regularly every evening for two weeks. The mother was given a telephone number and felt able to contact the nurses if she had any worries about the care or treatment of the child.

The child objected to the injection and fought with her parents on each occasion, creating considerable stress within the family. Administering the injection required one person to hold the child down while the other gave the injection. The father came home from work in his supper break to help, which was distressful for both him and the child. Finally, through a friend, the mother learnt about epi-syringes (which have a much smaller needle, give a more concentrated dose requiring less fluid, and can be used with one hand). The mother asked the consultant if he could supply her with this type of syringe as it would enable her to give the injection unaided, allowing her husband to take his break at work. The consultant knew nothing about the syringe and refused to pursue the request. The mother then approached the nurses, who had not heard of it, thought it sounded useful and wished the mother luck in trying to obtain it.

Through her friend, the mother contacted a specialist nurse in a specialist hospital some 50 miles away. This nurse visited the mother at home, supplied the syringe and needles, and wrote to the consultant, GP and community children's nurses explaining what she had done, indicating the change in prescription required. The specialist nurse also gave the mother information leaflets and a video demonstrating how to use the syringe, which the child watched repeatedly as it included other children talking about how much they had grown and demonstrated them having injections.

patient and family situations, and the behavioural responses to these situations. In those situations in which nurses have not been enabled to influence decision making, nursing care will, however, inevitably be unresponsive to patient and family need. Consequently, the holistic understanding necessary to integrate formal and informal care will not be available to those taking the decisions about service provision. The frontier will indeed appear impenetrable.

Vignette 3 illustrates how, in order to respond to problems, some nurses have developed the skills to counteract established practices and organisational boundaries when the need arises. In this case, the specialist nurse could have contacted staff locally with the information about the syringe and encouraged them to pass it onto the mother, but she could not be sure that this would happen. Instead, she supplied the syringe directly herself, using her time and some equipment that belonged to a hospital different from the one treating the mother, albeit still part of the NHS. This demonstrates how, in solving care problems, nurses become adept at diplomatically and effectively nego-tiating organisational boundaries within a care-as-ethical-position framework of provision based on individual problem solving. When policy analysts identify the need for 'seamless care', they rarely describe what it would look like in practice. This is one example that highlights how seamless care cuts across established contractual arrangements and accountability structures, and in so doing illustrates the complexi-ties associated with this type of provision.

Vignette 4 again demonstrates the biopsychosocial dimensions of nursing and highlights how the patient/family problem is only adequately resolved when all three dimensions are taken into account. The problem that the patient was experiencing with her parents only became visible when her parents visited; the patient did not disclose it to any staff. Although the parents were aware of the problem, they did not approach the nurses for help. The continuous care provided by the nurses meant that they inevitably observed the problem and were alerted to the difficulty. In a situation of non-disclosure, considerable skill was required to initiate communication about the problem. The ward sister had the necessary skills and was able to resolve the dilemma. In doing so, however, she had to keep the patient in hospital for an extra five or six days. In this situation, sufficient decision-making authority was vested in her post to enable her to do this, and thus she was able to accomplish her care.

Vignette 4 illustrates work for health undertaken by nurses; here, a care-as-therapeutic-relationship seemed to dominate the ward sister's action, and the outcome sought was a growth in understanding on the part of both the patient and her parents in order to reach a reconciliation that would enable them to resume their lives. Some elements of care-as-ethical-position are also demonstrated in that the ward sister individualised the length of stay in order to resolve the problem.

Vignette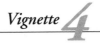

Resolving family guilt over an abortion

This incident involved a young teenage girl who had been admitted to a gynaecology ward following a privately undertaken abortion (Procter, 1989b). Subsequent to the abortion, the girl had developed a pelvic infection, and this was the reason for her admission to hospital. During the course of her admission, it quickly became apparent that the abortion had caused considerable trauma within her family. Her parents visited her regularly, but the daughter refused to see them or to speak to them. During discussion with the ward sister, the parents thought that this was because their daughter was angry with them as they had insisted on the abortion and they felt that they had overridden their daughter's wishes. On discussion with the daughter, it emerged that this was indeed the case, but this had nothing to do with the reason why she was refusing to see or speak to her parents. The reason was that she felt ashamed of her behaviour and was having difficulty admitting this to her parents. The level of emotional tension in the family was very high, and consequently it took several days for the full story to emerge and a few more days before the differences between the patient and her parents could be resolved. The ward sister acted throughout as a mediator between the patient and her parents. With the full support of the consultant, she decided to keep the patient in hospital until the tension in the family had been resolved. This she was successfully able to do, facilitating a full reconciliation between the patient and her parents. Only when she was completely satisfied that this had been achieved did the ward sister discharge the patient. From a strictly physiological point of view, the patient could have been discharged within 24 hours. From a psychological and emotional point of view, however, it took nearly a week for the ward sister to win the trust of the patient and to resolve the tension in the family surrounding the abortion.

The ethics of care and decision making in nursing

Vignettes 1–4 illustrate a number of dimensions of nursing in relation to ethics and decision making. Vignette 1 illustrates the familiar consequences of excluding the patient and nurses from decision-making processes altogether. The problems of caring identified in the previous chapter, of manipulation, coercion and guarded alliance, are all that are left when all parties are rendered powerless to affect the situation and produce a more positive outcome.

In the other three vignettes, both nurses and patients were proactive and facilitated to influence the decision-making process, the outcome being more positive. In each case, however, the decisions taken required nurses to negotiate across organisational boundaries or alter the level of service provision, thus committing resources in ways that did not necessarily reflect established funding streams or costed packages of provision.

In reviewing the literature on ethical decision making in nursing, Kuhse (1997) highlights a contemporary debate between feminist writers such as Gilligan (1982) and Noddings (1984), and traditional ethicists whose work can be traced back to the time of Socrates. According to Gilligan (1982), there are two moral 'languages'. The first is the historical language of impartiality or justice, which is regarded as the highest level of morality within traditional approaches to ethical reasoning. The second is an emerging language of 'care', which is premised on a world of relationships and psychological truths, in which an awareness of the connection between people gives rise to a recognition of responsibility for one another. In her formulation of the distinction between an ethics of 'impartiality' and an ethics of 'care', Gilligan aligns the former with a male, and the latter with a female, approach to justice.

Noddings (1984), Whitbeck (1984), Ruddick (1989) and Held (1993) have all suggested that the ethics of care ascribed to women arises from the work or functions typically performed by women, and by the fact that women have largely functioned in the 'private sphere' of the home and family, providing physical and emotional care for those with whom they have personal and/or lifelong relationships. Men, on the other hand, have largely worked in the 'public sphere', dealing with people to whom they are not personally related and with whom they develop instrumental and short-term relationships.

Kuhse (1997) accepts that this distinction may well exist and derive from gendered experiences of being born either male or female. She cannot, however, accept that this distinction is determined at a biological level by gender. It is, therefore, likely to change according to differing gendered experiences of men and women in different cultures and over time.

Proponents of the care approach to ethics argue that, in emphasising impartiality and universal obligations to all those affected by our actions, it is frequently necessary to sacrifice the concerns of those for whom we care at a personal level. Noddings (1984), in her description of feminine ethics, dismisses ethics based on universal principles, rules and rights, suggesting instead an ethics that is based on 'human affective response'. She contends that it is only in the context of the relationship between carer and cared for that issues of morality and ethics can be resolved. Resolution at all other levels fails to respond adequately to the particular features of a situation and can result in grave and unjustifiable injuries at this level.

Kuhse (1997), in her critique of Noddings, suggests that this approach is highly problematic: not only does it ignore power relations between the two parties, but it also results in arbitrary and parochial decision making. As Noddings herself notes, an ethics based on caring relationships displays a characteristic variability, and the care ethicist acts in a 'non-rulebound' fashion.

Kuhse (1997) draws a distinction between disobeying rules or instructions because one is opposed to them in principle and acting in a non-rulebound fashion. She suggests that nurses are fully justified in carrying out doctor's instructions when they know the instruction to be correct. In these circumstances, nurses are acting autonomously in the best interests of the patient rather than in a subservient role. In situations in which the nurse has a principled and knowledgeable objection to an instruction, the nurse is, however, entitled to question the instruction and has a moral right to refuse to carry it out. Similarly, Kuhse highlights numerous situations in which doctors would be correct in following nursing advice. Most of these situations derive from the nurses' more detailed understanding of the situation and, therefore, their ability to particularise decision making within the care context. Vignette 4 above is an example of this. Here, the medical staff left the decisions surrounding the discharge of the patient from hospital to the nursing staff.

Unlike Noddings, however, Kuhse suggests that these decisions need not be capricious, arbitrary, parochial or non-rulebound. Instead, Kuhse regards impartiality as an essential element of any adequate ethical approach. Indeed, she suggests that a truly impartial ethics would not be gender blind but would take account of gendered experiences in developing universal ethical principles.

This debate seems to be important for nursing particularly with the evolution of care-as-ethical-position paradigm. As Kuhse (1997) notes, nurses do not have a monopoly on caring behaviours. However, the structural features of their relationship with patients, in particular their provision of 24-hour care, or their remit to cover the 24-hour life space of the patient in assessing care provision, provides nurses with a unique perspective on the situation and a unique opportunity to observe the situation as it unfolds over time. The nurse in Vignette 2 above was not with the parents throughout the 24-hour period, but she needed to be satisfied that the parents could manage successfully until her next visit, or that adequate back-up and support were available if required. Similarly, the specialist nurse in Vignette 3 understood the daily stress experienced by the family in trying to give the injection and took specific action to ameliorate the problem.

In thinking about the 24-hour management of care, nurses are actively engaging with the dilemmas of care that occur at the interface between formal and informal care provision. The above discussion suggests that an understanding of the complexities of issues at the boundaries of formal and informal care can be gained from a close analysis of nursing work at this boundary. This analysis is strengthened by theoretical developments in nursing that have moved nursing from a care-as-duty position to that of knowledgeable practitioner.

Nurses solve problems in the context of the caring situation and in so doing make ethical and therapeutic decisions that incorporate biopsychosocial dimensions of health. In solving these problems, nurses frequently take principled decisions that cut across organisational boundaries and structures or alter the flow of resources to the patient within the care pathway, thus using resources differently from the initial streams to which they were committed. It is precisely this type of flexible response that care-as-communal-action (described by Bulmer, 1987) seeks to achieve. It follows that the expertise of nurses in solving these types of problem has a major contribution to make in planning for effective care in the community.

The role of reciprocity between nurses in accomplishing care

The above description of the role of the nurse as managing the 24-hour life space of the patient creates the need for a 24-hour structure of care provision. In the previous chapter, it was suggested that 24-hour responsibility for care also characterises the lives of many carers in the domestic arena. Here, it was recognised that, for a primary carer to be freed up to undertake non-caring activities, arrangements for secondary care had to be in place. Any failure in the secondary care arrangement or any change of circumstances that meant that the secondary carer could not provide appropriate cover pulled the primary carer back into the caring role. This reciprocal arrangement can also be found in nursing, as the following examples illustrate.

Vignette 5

Reciprocity in caring: covering another nurse's shift

A qualified nurse was undertaking a post-registration degree in nursing. She arrived 10 minutes late for a tutorial one day, clearly flustered and breathless. She explained that today was her day off, but her colleague had rung up to say that her son was sick and she could not get to work. The student agreed to cover the shift, which entailed arranging last minute child care for her own son, completing the shift, picking her son up, dropping him at home with his father and then travelling to the university for her tutorial.

Amazement was expressed that she had managed to turn up for the tutorial at all. The nurse said the degree was important and she did not want to miss anything. When asked how she felt about covering her colleague's shift, she said that she did not mind as her colleague's son was very ill with a childhood illness, that would eventually result in his death. The stress of this had contributed to the breakdown of her colleague's marriage, so she was on her own. Playing devil's advocate, it was suggested that if her colleague had a son who was that poorly, surely it would be better if she did not work. The student replied that her colleague's son was inevitably going to die and if her colleague gave up work, she would have nothing after he died; work was essential to ensure that she had a life afterwards.

The student went on to say that she did not mind helping her colleague out, especially as her own son was healthy and consequently she did not need to take time off work to look after him, which was a bonus. She finished by saying that, of course, if she ever did need a day off for her family or her studies, her colleague would always cover for her if she could.

In Vignette 5, the description of the nurse's day and the rationale given for her actions mirrored in almost every detail the classic text on social policy written by Richard Titmuss (1970). *The Gift Relationship: From Human Blood to Social Policy.* In this text, Titmuss uses the blood transfusion service as an analogy for a collective social insurance policy whereby people give when they are healthy in order to receive when they are sick, recognising that to give blood freely and never require a transfusion is the preferred situation for most blood donors, but if they ever needed a blood transfusion, or for those who did, it would be there. In the case described in Vignette 5, a similar reciprocal relationship is described whereby the student willingly gave up her day off knowing that she might never claim it back directly but knowing that it would be available if she needed it. She also recognised that her colleague's need for a flexible system of managing her time off was so much greater than her own because her colleague's situation was so much more tragic. That her own child was healthy and that she did not have the same problem rendered the odd extra unpaid day at work insignificant in comparison.

The action of the student and the rationale she gave in many ways embody the key characteristics of nursing as health work. In thinking through the problem, she recognised the long-term needs of her colleague over the short-term demands of her son's illness and the hospital's requirement for a nurse to cover a shift. By covering her shift, the student was, therefore, nursing her colleague, enabling her in turn to nurse her son.

Gould (1984) similarly highlights reciprocity as a liberating form of social relationship. She proposes that, when individuals act with respect to each other, their relationships take the form either of domination and subordination or of reciprocity. Reciprocity, Gould argues, presupposes equality in that it recognises that the other person is an equally free agent consenting to the relationship. In its most highly developed state, Gould maintains reciprocal relationships go beyond equality and acknowledge the differences of the other in terms of the other's own projects and goals.

This layered and multidimensional pattern of relationships is reflective of the discussion of the key features of caring work given in the previous chapter. It is not however, a unique case. Examples of nurses working in this way were found in a recent investigation of the work of community children's nurses (ENB, 1999). In this, community children's nurses recognised the need of parents looking after sick children at home to have 24-hour access to a nursing service. A wide variety of arrangements were introduced by nurses, often independently of management and of commissioning agencies, which enabled them to meet this need and accommodate it within the demands of their own domestic lives.

A similar scenario is given by Poole (1998), in which she describes the setting up of a small community nursing team attached to a fund-holding general practice. Here, she suggests 'the team covers its own members' off-duty time including sickness and holidays' (Poole, 1998, p. 61). The above scenarios illustrate how nurses, who are frequently primary carers in their domestic lives, can develop patterns of work organisation that enable them successfully to manage both roles simultaneously.

The way in which nurses accomplish this is via a very sophisticated system of reciprocity set up by the nurses themselves, which enables them to cover both their domestic and their professional commitments. Personal sickness is only one reason, often a very minor reason in the whole list of events that require nurses to take time off from work. Other reasons include the care of their own children with coughs, colds and general and occasionally serious childhood ailments, the care of elderly relatives when sick or in need, and attendance at school ceremonies, plays, assemblies and so on. Together, the activities associated with the care and nurture of their own families may well dominate reasons for non-attendance at work. Personal sickness may be a minor event compared with the more prevalent and pressing demands of their families.

Nurses, in interweaving domestic and work commitments, can set up complex systems of reciprocity to manage both formal and informal caring. An illness requiring a child to be kept home from school can, for example, be responded to by a series of telephone calls in which the nurse, staying home to look after her child, reallocates her day's work to the other nurses, who in turn reorganise their day in order to incorporate this work. The other nurses respond because the ability to respond is a feature of nursing work and the next week it might be their child who was sick so they would need to call in the favour. As nurses, they understand the unpredictable nature of illness as experienced at an individual level and assume that few nurses choose to have a sick child or to keep a child unnecessarily home from school.

The total workload in nursing is, therefore, covered not individually but collectively. Nurses frequently do not claim additional wages for covering this extra work; they do it so that when they unexpectedly need time off, they too can be confident that their patients will be cared for. Managing caring requires systems that are sensitive and responsive to the complex and unpredictable demands that characterise this work both formally and informally. Nurses have repeatedly demonstrated their ability to implement organic, flexible working practices. However, these practices frequently fail to fit with bureaucratic control systems that demand excessive planning and monitoring (James, 1994). The frequent disputes that arise in nursing around time off in lieu of hours worked is an example of a lack of fit between the two systems.

Joshi (1991), in a discussion of sex and motherhood in the labour market, has illustrated how the dual characteristic of being a female and a mother leads to discrimination in the labour market. She calls for the development of 'family-friendly policies' that would recognise the caring work of women in the home and provide support for this. These policies would reduce the seclusion of those being cared for and their carers from the adult environment and thus seek to reduce the tension between the individual and the family. In so doing, they would present families with more resources and more options to protect the weak and dependent without penalising the carers. The organic and flexible working practices developed by nurses provide models for this type of approach. They recognise the need to integrate care-as-labour with care-as-communal-action. This legitimises attendance at school plays and assemblies, as well as time off to care for sick children and elderly relatives, as part of a rounded community, not one starved of most of its adult inhabitants during office hours. Nursing operates throughout the 24-hour period so scheduling nursing to accommodate these needs, while certainly complex, should not be thwarted by an overly bureaucratic approach dominated by a 9–5 mentality.

In order to accomplish these flexible working arrangements, nurses take numerous particularistic ethical decisions, some of which are contrary to established policies and procedures. These decisions enable them both to prioritise between and to integrate their formal and informal caring roles. In so doing, nurses are accepting individual accountability for the care of their patients but recognising that this care is delivered collectively in much the same way that parents manage the 24-hour care of their children, particularly those of school age.

There are a large number of women employed in nursing and health care. The employment of women and their dual role as workers and domestic carers is not a small marginal problem for the NHS but a major issue for the smooth running of organisations and, ultimately, society. Recent high-profile political debates on the pivotal role of the family and the erosion of this role in post-industrial society reflect this concern. A failure to recognise the duality of role and life experience gives rise to a narrow view of health care as being similar to that provided by the health service. In reality, most care is provided outside the health and social services, frequently by the same people who work for these services. To ignore the impact of this on health and social service organisations puts up artificial and unreal barriers that people in their daily lives negotiate with increasing degrees of frustration and time wasting.

The distinction between formal and informal care, which permeates social policy literature, creates a duality in which formal service providers are regarded in every way as being distinctive from informal providers of care. In fact, most people involved in providing formal care simultaneously provide informal care in their domestic lives. In order to accomplish this, they are in turn dependent on an array of secondary care supports from childminders to schools to the extended family. Rarely, however, is this taken into account when planning and commissioning service provision.

Developing responsive management

James (1994) has charted the management theories that have dominated health care provision in the UK over the past 50 years. Her work illustrates how the government has attempted to control health care delivery through the dual forces of bureaucracy and the imposition of a market economy. Neither approach, she argues, was successful because they disempowered both professionals and service users alike. James identifies three modes of service delivery for the future:

1. *the professional bureaucracy*, in which organisations are led by people recognised as professional experts, who carry extensive credibility in the organisation;

2. *the market organisation*, which interprets the service as a business in which decisions are negotiated rather than imposed;

3. *the network organisation*, a new and emergent form of organisation characterised by a commitment to the community rather than the organisation, which perceives its business as enabling and works by investing authority in others and by empowerment.

The coping management described by Davies (1992), discussed in the last chapter as being characteristic of the ineffectiveness of nurse managers, shares some of the features of the network organisation. The management behaviour displayed by nurses and described by Davies reflects a particular set of values that includes meeting the needs of patients and putting the interest of patients before all other considerations, including the specific goals of the organisation. According to James (1994, p. 104), people who flourish in network organisations 'are those who can hold onto an image of connectedness without necessarily needing the superstructure of buildings or of professional identity to hold them together. Regulation comes from the user, in the form of quality assurance and participation'. Nursing, in its evolved form as care-as-ethical-position, reflects many of these dimensions, as exemplified in Vignettes 2–5 above.

From this perspective even the use of the terms 'dysfunctional behaviour' and 'coping management' (Davies, 1992) become problematic. Such terms still locate the problem with nurses' behaviour and their inability to make demands on behalf of themselves and their profession in order to reduce the stress level and increase the power and status of nursing. A more constructive approach to the problem might be to locate nursing management behaviour in the arena of values. Here the coping strategies used by nurses gain credibility as organisations move from bureaucratic and professional forms of control to control centred on problem solving and connecting with other organisations and the needs of patients (Walby *et al.*, 1994).

Integrating caring work into organisational structures

As described in the previous chapter, care is a universal construct. Philosophically, the term is used to define our humanity, and a consciousness of collective care is used to distinguish us from other species. In practice, however, care-as-labour is dislocated from mainstream organisational activities and located primarily with women in the domestic arena, and nurses and other predominantly female care workers in health care. The shared features of care-as-labour means that many attributes of informal care derived from the affective domain, including particularistic ethical decision making, connectedness between feelings and action, and the use of concepts of caring to distinguish what matters in a given situation, are also features of nursing.

Care-as-labour is frequently viewed as drudgery, hard work and expensive, if done properly. This dominant view of care work is reflective of care-as-duty, which, as this chapter demonstrates, arises when decision-making opportunities are denied to carers. The adoption of the care-as-duty paradigm fails to acknowledge the ethical resolution of problems arising out of the everyday practice of caring.

Denying the decision-making component of caring practices can give rise to arbitrary, capricious and in some cases apparently callous decisions. The caring ethics proposed by Gilligan (1982) and Noddings (1984) highlights the importance of particularising decision making in caring situations to prevent callousness. The challenge, however, is to do this in a way that simultaneously supports ethical impartiality (Kuhse, 1997), an intellectual challenge that goes to the core of contemporary policy issues, as depicted by Bulmer (1987) and Twigg (1989). When nurses are able to problem solve within the caring situation, they can exercise considerable elegance in integrating formal and informal care and in so doing resolving difficult ethical decisions.

If we return to the debates described in Chapter 3, it is apparent that the main challenges facing health care organisations are (i) how to increase the number of disability-free life years, and (ii) how to facilitate the inclusion of people suffering from disabilities into mainstream society. These challenges will not be met in hospitals, but in primary and community care. Chapter 3 also indicated that the biggest cost facing health care providers arises not from the provision of care work or even from the ageing of the population but from the spiralling costs associated with medical technology, in particular the ineffective use of this technology.

In striving to accommodate the spiralling cost of technology, other aspects of provision are frequently undercut; nursing in particular seems to be particularly susceptible to such downward pressures (McKenna, 1995; McKee *et al.*, 1998). This chapter argues that women's failure to access high-status positions reflects not a deficit in their ability but the additional complexity of their lives, derived from their dual role. This is currently viewed as a handicap and something to be overcome (Joshi, 1991). The argument being advanced here is that, far from being a handicap, the understanding that women derive from their experiences of their dual role has a critical contribution to make in shaping more holistic, integrated and humanistic solutions to organisational and social problems. This does not derive from the experiences of being female but from the experiences of juggling the demands of two roles, a worker role and a domestic role, which are often viewed as incompatible. Only by developing organisational processes that make these roles compatible can the necessary skills and the insight be bought to bear on the complex human problem of caring.

The concerns of nurses as carers could, if their voice were listened to, provide a brake on the pursuit of technological and instrumental solutions to human problems generated by male approaches to work and problem solving derived from specialist, individualistic and single-minded approaches to knowledge production. The development of 'family-friendly policies' suggested by Joshi (1991) becomes more than just a plea for equality. It reflects a realisation that if we are to use medical technology responsibly and effectively, this can only be achieved by integrating it with the everyday needs and concerns of the people using the technology rather than the other way round. Care-as-ethical-position provides a theoretical framework for exploring how this can be achieved. Nurses, both academically and in practice, have made a considerable intellectual contribution to the development of care-as-ethical-position, and this contribution needs to be recognised in developing people- and family-centred health care organisations.

An understanding and integration of caring into mainstream organisational and economic thinking could have profound repercussions on the type of knowledge produced and the solutions identified by this knowledge. This could be critical in curbing the tendency for health care to promote tertiary solutions to health care problems based on resource-intensive technological developments. The concerns of caring, with its emphasis on long-term goals rather than short-term technological expediency, could be a powerful conceptual model for producing more sustainable solutions to contemporary health care problems. But the voice of people struggling to manage roles that are currently viewed as incompatible must first be heard, without denying the experience of these two roles. For as soon as the experience is denied, the potential contribution is lost.

Summary and conclusion

This chapter illustrates how nurses operate at the margins of informal and formal care, mediating between informal carers on the one hand and the power brokers within service provision on the other. Nurses contend with the interface between formal and informal care personally as well as professionally. The majority of nurses are female, and many will simultaneously pursue informal and family caring roles alongside their formal professional role. Given this position, the transformational power of the role is formidable. Nurses have the potential to transform both local communities and the use of power in providing services for those communities.

The role is, however, complex. If nursing moves too far into alignment with the power brokers, it loses its connectedness to communities. If it moves too closely in with communities, it becomes disenfranchised from local power bases. Much of the nursing behaviour described by Davies (1992) has to be understood as a manifestation of the contradictions and paradoxes associated with maintaining a vital marginal transformational role. If nurses adopt too many characteristics associated with the effective use of power, their ability to work effectively with the disempowered is compromised. If nurses adopt too many characteristics of informal affective care, they do not appear to operate effectively within a rational-legal organisational environment. Embracing this role and understanding these paradoxes may help nurses to come to terms with their position in health care, and may also help others to understand why nurses do not always adopt the behaviours deemed appropriate for the role.

Chapter 6

Accomplishing Caring in Multi-professional, Multi-agency Settings

The previous chapter demonstrated the centrality of caring to understanding and tackling some of the major challenges facing health care organisations today. This chapter reviews caring within the context of multiprofessional, multi-agency service delivery. It continues the theme introduced in Chapter 4 that caring is a universal phenomenon rather than an aspect of care delivery that can be claimed by any one professional group or agency. Certain features of caring, especially the work associated with care-as-labour, have, however, been devolved to specific groups of workers, in particular nurses, nursery nurses and residential care workers. Unqualified staff such as health care assistants and care workers in the community perform much of this work.

Nursing has been privileged by access to higher education and research. It has also retained professional responsibility for the delivery of physical and emotional care to patients, as described in the previous chapter. As a consequence, nursing is in a position to develop a body of knowledge on the delivery of this type of care that could inform the resolution of policy dilemmas associated with promoting health and integrating people with disabilities into mainstream communal activities. This chapter reviews the evolution of this body of knowledge on the development of care-as-communal-action.

Care-as-communal-action

In describing care-as-communal-action Bulmer (1987) highlights the variations and overlaps between statutory, commercial, voluntary and informal forms of care. Drawing on the work of Litwak and Szelenyi

(1969), he highlights three different types of care that can be provided in the community:

1. *physical care, tending* and *help with personal finances*, which is most usually provided by family and close kin. If this source of support is not available, formal carers such as care assistants, nurses or social workers are called in;

2. *face-to-face contact* with neighbours, which are most suited to emergencies and activities that require daily observation but are relatively undemanding;

3. *friendship ties*, which involve an element of choice from both parties and can be used to reduce social isolation.

As Bulmer notes, these three forms of care in the community are not easily substituted for each other. In developing care in the community, the type of care provided and who provides it are, therefore, critical issues.

Bulmer's discussion of care-as-communal-action focuses on meeting the individual care needs of people living in the community. In discussing the concept of the community, Bulmer recognises the difficulties of defining this term. Communities can be characterised by anonymity and isolation. People may not identify with their neighbours, nor may they feel any allegiance or solidarity with them.

Tilden and Weinert (1987, p. 614) distinguish between social support and social networks. They describe social networks as 'the structural inter-relationships of family, friends, neighbours, co-workers, and others who provide support'. Social networks are characterised by dimensions such as 'size, density (the extent to which people in the network know each other), frequency of contact, durability or length of relationships and homogeneity (the similarity of people in the network)' (Tilden and Weinhert, 1987, p. 614). Social support refers to the psychosocial and tangible support provided by the social network and received by the person. It comprises emotional support (love, trust, concern and care); appraisal support (feedback, constructive criticism and affirmation of self-worth); informational support (advice and information); and instrumental support (reciprocal child care arrangements, loans and financial support).

The link between the level and quality of social support, and an individual's and/or family's resilience to adversity, is the subject of considerable research. Stewart and Tilden (1995) highlight evidence suggesting that integration into a social network and the ability to draw resources from that network have been identified as factors that protect health and promote physical recovery from illness.

Antonovsky (1996, p. 15) has posed the question 'What explains the movement toward the health pole of the health disease/dis-ease continuum?' In his search for an answer to this question, he has identified what he calls 'generalised resistance resources'. This refers to the characteristics of an individual or group (family) that facilitate successful coping with the inherent stressors of human existence. Antonovsky's work indicates that a range of social and psychological factors predispose towards the development of generalised resistance resources; these include wealth, ego strength, social support and cultural stability, all of which promote health (Antonovsky, 1993). As Antonovsky (1996) notes, the concept of resilience is closely related to, and shares many characteristics with, the concept of coping.

Lazarus (1992) has highlighted the centrality of a person's coping responses to his or her effective adaptation to illness and disability. He poses a question similar to that of Antonovsky, suggesting that 'the central question in coping is a complex one, namely, *which forms of coping, in which persons,* and *under which conditions* result in positive and negative short- and long-term adaptational outcomes?' (Lazarus, 1992, p. 11). While Antonovsky's work focused on life history and the development of resilience over time, Lazarus, however, focused on the facilitation of coping behaviours following the onset of chronic illness. He concludes that each illness has its own unique source of psychological stress, some of which is shared with other illnesses. He suggests therefore, that the coping process we should encourage will depend on:

- the person's appraisal of meaning;
- the person's coping style and the stage of the illness;
- the fact that general strategies of stress management might succeed with some and fail with others;
- the best intervention involving a careful assessment of the appraisal and coping variables for each patient, taking into account personal agendas, circumstances, illness, prognosis and life stage;
- listening to the patient carefully, discovering his or her sources of threat, harm and distress.

The factors listed by Lazarus reflect the work of Antonovsky in that they highlight the importance of learning about individuals' life histories and characteristic coping strategies in order to identify how best to help them to cope with illness. As Lazarus points out, this is something that is almost absent in medical practice, namely a great concern for and awareness of the patient's emotional life.

The work of Lazarus (1992), Antonovsky (1993, 1996) and Stewart and Tilden (1995) illustrates the interconnections between the public domain of social structures, environments and communities, and the private domain of family relationships, roles and responsibilities. Public policy, however, remains reticent about breaching the public/private boundary. The chief medical officer in the UK has recognised that the ability to improve an individual's health 'is inextricably linked with their social, environmental and economic circumstances and the health and other public services available to them' (Chief Medical Officer, 1998, p. 9). The report acknowledges that to deliver the right service to local people at the time it is needed requires health, social services, other parts of local government and voluntary agencies to work together in partnership.

The HAZ initiative, introduced into the UK, is designed to facilitate partnerships between 'the NHS, local authorities, community groups and the voluntary and business sectors to develop and implement a health strategy to deliver within their area measurable improvements in public health and in the outcomes and quality of treatment and *care*' (DoH, 1998a, p. 10, emphasis added).

In order to achieve these partnerships, HAZs are able to pool budgets between all public sector providers in order to undertake the joint commissioning and delivery of services. HAZs are also able to transfer funds between agencies and delegate functions to one another. For example, the NHS will be able to provide social care services, and social services will be able to provide a limited range of community health services, such as chiropody or community physiotherapy, beyond the level possible under current powers.

The opportunity to develop partnerships for the commissioning and delivery of services recognises the importance of actively involving the public and local communities in shaping service provision. It is derived from a public health perspective that seeks to promote health by creating healthy living environments, which enable social integration (Ashton and Seymour, 1988). The example of the Peckham experiment (Ashton, 1992) is often cited to illustrate the close links between personal health promotion and social and environmental living conditions.

The HAZ focuses primarily on the boundaries between interagency provision and in this sense promotes a more systemic, integrated approach to provision. However, in taking the HAZ initiative forward, the critical issues surrounding care-as-physical-labour and the provision of such care is merged with wider agendas focusing on social and environmental determinants of health. The complex ethical issues surrounding the provision of care-as-physical-labour, in particular the policy concerns arising at the boundaries of formal and informal care provision, are in danger of being delegated to families and unqualified care workers and consequently marginalised from the mainstream public health agenda. The HAZ agenda cannot claim to promote holistic health (see Chapter 2 for a definition of holistic health) as it has not clarified the issues surrounding the integration of the individualistic approach to health, which predominates in health care, with the social model of health, which informs public health policy.

The difficulties confronting the resolution of problems at an individual level are illustrated in Vignette 6, subtitled Leanne's story. Twenty years later, are we any closer to meeting the needs of vulnerable people such as Leanne? The following issues arise from Leanne's story and can be seen to dominate contemporary health and social care policy.

Prevention

The Health of the Nation target E1 aims to reduce the death rate for accidents among children aged under 15 by at least 33 per cent over the period 1990 to 2005. What is to be prevented here in the case of Leanne – the initial fire that caused the burns, the recurrence of the contractures following skin grafting, the future awaiting Leanne of child prostitution, teenage pregnancies, drug addiction, the cycle, in fact, of deprivation, of which she was so clearly an example? And what of *her* children?

Resources

Many resources went into the care of Leanne, but it is questionable whether they were used appropriately, whether their use was effective or efficient, or just a waste of time. That this use of resources could be legitimised by appeal to medical needs was, however, never questioned. Using the same (in cost terms) resources differently was never even considered. The concepts underpinning HAZs are concerned with using resources differently and more effectively. At the same time as introducing HAZs, the government in the UK has declared that it 'is committed to the historic principle that if you are ill or injured there will be a national health service there to help you; and access to it will be based on need and need alone' (DoH, 1998c, p. 4).

The case of Leanne highlights the complexity of delivering integrated care that meets all of her many-faceted needs for health (in the fullest sense, as discussed in Chapter 2) rather than just the more obvious biomedical need associated with the skin graft. While access to the skin graft is relatively uncontentious within the principles of the

---

Vignette **6**

Leanne's story

The author experienced this incident when she was a student nurse, over 20 years ago. The incident concerns a child – Leanne – who was about 10 years old. She had been admitted to the paediatric ward for a skin graft to both armpits, which were severely contracted following extensive deep burns she had received to her chest and back after she had set fire to her own night-dress a few years previously. The burns were completely healed, but she was unable to raise her arms above her head, hence the need for skin grafting.

Leanne lived in a hotel room in Kings Cross, London, with numerous brothers and sisters who all shared the same bed as her. Her mother was a prostitute and did not visit Leanne the whole time she was in hospital. Leanne's behaviour on the ward was less than sociable. She was incredibly aggressive to the staff and to the other children, frequently biting, kicking and hitting anyone who upset her, which was easily done. What is more, Leanne's language was foul, and her use of sexual expletives was beyond any range that I had ever encountered before. She was extremely sexually promiscuous, making lewd sexual suggestions and advances to the male medical staff, porters or indeed any man who entered the ward, including the fathers of some of the other children.

Despite all of this, the operation went ahead and the skin grafting was performed. Following the operation, plaster casts were made, into which Leanne had to be strapped for up to 12 hours each day. These casts kept her arms raised up above her head to prevent the contractures recurring as the skin grafts healed. The task – and it was a task – of strapping Leanne into the plaster cast each day was delegated to the most inexperienced member of the nursing staff, usually a student or pupil nurse, and failing that an auxiliary. Leanne did not react well to this cast. If anyone ever managed to withstand the violence associated with putting it on to Leanne, their efforts were in vain because, despite the difficulties, she somehow managed to wriggle out of it within minutes.

Vignette 6

Leanne's story (cont'd)

Daily, the student nurses, along with the auxiliaries, struggled with Leanne and her cast, and daily we failed. On one occasion, rather than strap Leanne into the cast, I started to clear out an ancient, dusty and very deep cupboard in the corner of the ward. It was filled with an array of broken toys and discarded bits of equipment. At the back of the cupboard were some old books that I had learnt to read with at school. I was aware that the books had since been condemned as sexist, but started to flick through them, noticing Leanne watching me. I told her about the books and explained the debate surrounding them. I gave her a book and asked her to tell me what she thought. Then I realised that she could not read. At the same time as I realised this she realised that I had found out, and I could tell she was deeply ashamed. In some clumsy way, I managed to reassure her that I did not think it was anything to be ashamed about. We took the books over to her bed and I sat down with her behind the curtains and started to teach her to read. We struck up a deal; you wear the plaster cast, and I'll teach you to read. No one else noticed what was going on; they were just relieved that Leanne was out of the way and occupied. We kept this going for the next few days until one day I came on duty to find that Leanne had been summarily discharged. She was to continue to wear the cast at night in a bed that she shared with her numerous brothers and sisters in a hotel room in Kings Cross.

NHS, enabling Leanne to benefit from the services provided by the NHS raises a host of controversial and ethically difficult issues. In delivering integrated care to meet all her health care needs, the frontier between formal and informal care, between statutory provision and the autonomy of families to manage their own affairs, becomes a central, contentious and negotiated aspect of service delivery.

The work of Abel-Smith (1994) discussed in Chapter 3 provided a description of hospitals as being increasingly focused on the provision of high-technology medicine to diagnose and treat sophisticated physiological problems. Such technology is expensive to develop and purchase, and requires highly trained personnel to maintain and use it. This interpretation of hospital provision assumes that patients are admitted to hospital because they require access to this level of technology. The vignettes above illustrate that concentrating on physiological needs independently of psychosocial problems undermines the efficient use of technology for patients with complex problems.

In Vignettes 6 and 7, the focus of hospital admission is the management of physical symptoms, yet the problems prompting admission to hospital and causing difficulties following discharge derive from a combination of social and psychological factors interacting with the physical symptoms to produce patient and carer stress. If the health service is to be successful, service provision needs to breach the frontier between formal and informal care responsibilities in order to break the cycle of stress demonstrated in these incidents. Co-ordinating service

---

Vignette 7

Legitimising anxiety as a need

This is the case of a 73-year-old man interviewed as part of a study into effective discharge from hospital (Pearson *et al.*, 1998). The patient had a history of chronic obstructive airways disease, angina, impaired function of his left ventricle, and prostate problems. He had lived alone since the death of his wife two years previously and received a comprehensive care package through Age Concern. His two adult sons and daughter lived close by. Since retirement, he had led a varied and active life, but with the progression of his various physical problems, he was becoming increasingly housebound. He viewed himself as independent and did not want to burden his children or move into residential care.

The patient had a history of frequent admission to hospital, often ringing for an ambulance rather than call his GP. The consultant in charge of the case commented that 'he came in [to hospital] because he wants to, because he worries and because he gets anxious about his condition'. The consultant suggested, 'He'll be back in hospital before his next outpatient appointment with either breathlessness or angina.' The district nurse looking after the patient was aware that the patient called an ambulance to gain admission to hospital and commented, 'He has lots of medical problems and he dwells over these endlessly... his life revolves around his medical problems.' The social worker commented, 'Well he has social services, he's got a caring family; however much care you gave this man it would never be enough, everything revolves around his illness. He put in a request last year for more home help and when asked what help he needed it was to cut his grass' (Pearson *et al.*, 1998, pp. 82–3).

provision is unlikely to provide practice models that resolve carers' needs and simultaneously promote effective self-care. To address these issues, service co-ordination needs to be accompanied by a shared theoretical understanding of the types of health outcome sought for patients and families, and by a shared ethical philosophy about how services integrate with informal family care to achieve health.

Individualised patient-centred care

The aim of much contemporary government policy is 'to put the needs of users and carers firmly at the centre of health and social service provision' (DoH, 1998c, p. 8). Vignettes 6 and 7 above, illustrate how, through practice, some of the most complex dilemmas facing policy makers are encountered. The discussion of ethical decision making in the previous chapter illustrated how an ethics of care as depicted by Gilligan (1982) and Noddings (1984) starts with the individual and evolves from a resolution of individual problems. It is connected and particularistic. This was contrasted with more traditional male-orientated approaches to ethics in which universal abstract ethical principles are applied impartially to a given situation.

In Vignette 6, the ethical principle of universal access to health care was upheld for Leanne. However, a holistic resolution of Leanne's total health care needs seems to require an understanding of and respect for her unique situation. The ethics-as-care philosophy implies that decisions should be made within the context of this situation and be designed to bring about a progressive resolution of her problems that would enable her to co-operate with and benefit from the skin grafting.

Similarly, in Vignette 7, the professionals seemed unable to address the fears and anxieties experienced by this patient in relation to his progressive symptoms. He remained isolated with his disease processes, which he talked about endlessly and yet failed to come to terms with. His frequent self-referral to hospital indicated that this type of provision was a chosen or preferred option for this patient, but it was considered an inappropriate response by those who provided the services. His request for a home help was assessed on tasks to be completed, which he felt obliged to identify. The use of abstract and generalisable criteria for accessing services forces this patient to emphasise physiological needs or tasks to be completed because of disability and consequently failed to enable him, or the professionals caring for him, to identify and address the true sources of anxiety experienced by this patient. This gave rise to successive requests for further help that were met with similarly ineffective responses.

The interpretation of the role of hospitals given by Abel-Smith (1994), and reinforced on a daily basis by the activities of numerous professional staff, contrasts sharply with the everyday use made of hospitals by many patients (Pearson *et al.*, 1998). Maintaining a technological interpretation of the role of hospitals compounds the patient's vulnerability within the situation while simultaneously reducing the work of hospitals to occupy a marginal and relatively ineffective role. An individual ethics of care such as that proposed by Gilligan (1982) would reinterpret the role of statutory agencies in intervening in these types of situation by encouraging a contextual, particularistic and situational understanding of individual need in order to inform service delivery. However, as Kuhse (1997) cautions, the ethics of care is highly contentious as it can give rise to decisions that appear to be capricious, parochial and arbitrary. Consequently, this approach requires considerable skill and expertise within a theoretical framework of care if these pitfalls are to be avoided.

A new practitioner to solve an old problem

In the UK, nursing is currently facing a plethora of new roles and opportunities encompassed under the scope of professional practice (UKCC, 1992) and giving rise to attempts to delineate specialist and advanced practice. Vignettes 6 and 7 above illustrate how very complex problems require not only the co-ordination of multiprofessional input, but also a clear theoretical and possibly holistic understanding of what it is that the services are trying to achieve in each case.

Ward and McMahon (1998), in attempting to develop services to meet the complex needs of children such as Leanne, describe the development of what they term 'therapeutic child care'. In developing this area, they recognise the extensive range of settings in which this practice is carried out, as well as the fact that the staff working in these settings do not necessarily identify themselves as coming under the same professional and conceptual umbrella. Some of the staff identify themselves as coming primarily from social work, others from nursing, others from special education and still others from group analysis or child psychotherapy. However, despite the diverse professional backgrounds, Ward and McMahon (1998, p. 3) suggest that:

across this wide range of settings could be found a large number of staff all attempting to achieve broadly the same therapeutic objectives with some deeply troubled young people and probably all needing to draw on each of the perspectives mentioned above.

Ward illustrates this process in his description of the care given to Peter, a four-year-old attending a day centre (see Vignette 8).

Vignette 8 illustrates the attention to detail and continuity of care necessary to resolve problems at an individual level. This example also shows how different members of the multiprofessional team were bought in to address the problem once the source of the problem had been identified. The knowledge and skills required to identify the source of the problem combined close observation, investigation, questioning, thinking and understanding from the child's perspective in the context of his daily ongoing behaviour and activities. Problem solving, therefore, required a knowledge of the 24-hour life space of the child and the opportunity to observe his behaviour over time in different

---

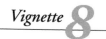

Vignette 8

Peter's story

It was noticed that Peter frequently became agitated shortly before the end of the day. For no apparent reason, he would often begin racing around the building, avoiding contact with adults, before eventually colliding with another child or object and collapsing in a heap crying. This behaviour was in contrast to his subdued and compliant behaviour during the rest of the day. His mother would not intervene but would end up shouting at him angrily after he had fallen and hurt himself.

His behaviour upset both staff and children, but no one intervened. Staff attempted to identify the reason for his behaviour, discussing it with his mother, who was unable to explain it. Eventually, a staff member recalled that another child described one of the drivers who escorted families home at the end of the day as 'Peter's daddy'. At a distance, Peter too had mistaken the driver for his absent father. This incident had gone unnoticed except by the other child and Peter's mother, who did not like to acknowledge that Peter was still attached to his father. Once this was recognised, it was addressed by a play therapist working with Peter, and his mother was given the opportunity to discuss her anxieties with a member of staff. (Ward and McMahon, 1998, pp. 3–4)

situations and contexts. Staff required the skill to link the child's behaviour with his concerns within his daily environment and understand how these concerns were linked to the wider social fabric of his life.

Much of this information is privileged family information and therefore, informal, private and inaccessible. Accessing such information in therapeutic environments recognises problems associated with family functioning and in this case required an understanding of the mother's difficulties in helping her child to accept the family situation in which he found himself.

Vignette 8 illustrates how different academic and theoretical perspectives are combined with the integration of practice arising from diverse professional groups, in order to resolve problems at an individual level as they arise in the context of care provision. This new and evolving form of care moves daily care forward from custodial care or care-as-duty towards the care-as-ethical-position described by Kitson (1993) and Benner and Wrubel (1989). It illustrates both the skill level required to provide this type of care and the sensitive nature of care provision, which is designed to work directly with the daily activities of families.

A similar form of care provision was recognised in a focus group held with representatives from a range of children's charities. The focus group formed part of larger study into the developing role of the community children's nurse (Procter *et al.*, 1998). During the focus group meeting, members described how the families of sick children with long-term disabilities required regular flexible help because they were worn out by the level of care they were frequently expected to provide. Some families were not, however, confident to let others provide this care. Members of the focus group suggested that what parents frequently wanted was someone to provide respite in other areas of their lives, rather than coming in to do the physiotherapy for example. The members of the charity focus group suggested that, in their experience, when this type of service was made available, parents did not actually make excessive demands on it, just as long as the service was provided on a regular basis and the parents could depend on it.

In discussing the level of competence required by someone to fill this helping role effectively, members of the focus group saw the need to develop a worker who was able to provide 'hands-on' support to the family in order to help with the daily management of the child and of other family members. The type of skill required was, however, seen to be problematic. Professional staff were considered to be overqualified for the role and unprepared to undertake some of the menial tasks associated with the role, for example, doing the ironing if this was the problem for the family.

On the other hand, some of the situations in which these workers could find themselves were very difficult and required high-level skills, for instance when working with families with a very challenging and complex set of needs, or when they had anxieties such as child abuse. As one member of the group commented:

> The people whom the families relate to best are probably the least highly qualified, because they have less or fewer problems about their own status. …Then I worry they might be under-trained, that is rather than under-qualified, because qualification is probably the least of it. It is training and experience. (Procter *et al.*, 1998 p. 136)

The members of the charities focus group were acutely aware of the stresses experienced by families in caring for sick children. The focus group highlighted how caring for a sick child can have an adverse impact on the interpersonal relationships within the family or, as one member put it, 'the parents' relationship is very often, literally falling apart' (Procter *et al.*, 1998 p. 136). This group member went on to describe how he was trying to find people who could work as family support workers while simultaneously helping the parents to address some of the problems in their relationship. He commented:

> we could somehow perhaps play some role in aiding the parents to recog- nise that, and perhaps, while the child is still alive, do something to stop the child's quality of life being severely undermined by the parents' being unable to control their emotions in front of the children… and we are slowly moving into this area, because it is quite difficult, each time that we recognise that there is a role for us there, we first obviously have to ask someone to help us do this; the second thing is that it is an expensive busi- ness, to raise the skill level of our staff. (Procter *et al.*, 1998, p. 136)

In this context, there was a discussion about the type of communica- tion skills required by someone undertaking a family support worker role. One member of the group had been involved in setting up a national vocational qualification (NVQ) course for counselling skills for family support workers. She commented:

> It is almost impossible because… psychodynamic people will not join with the cognitive therapists, who won't talk to the humanists who absolutely hate the Rogerians. It is very, very difficult, when what you are actually talking about is actually listening to what people are saying, actively listening I suppose. If one wants to be more precise about what that means and playing a role that actually enables that person to think out loud and to talk through for their own benefit and arrive at their own conclusions,

courses of action or inaction... That to me is the low-tech end that is most helpful to most officers [family support workers], and what we all tend to do is go down the specialist route. (Procter *et al.*, 1998 p. 137)

The discussion of the needs of families derived from the focus group of children's charities suggested that overqualification and specialisation led to the development of inappropriate skills. The group seemed to be suggesting that, for this type of work, it is perhaps misleading to develop hierarchies of skill based on increasing specialisation and the acquisition of increasing amounts of technical knowledge. Undertaking so-called 'low-tech' counselling might actually require considerable skill if it were to be effective.

A similar case for establishing 'something entirely new' was alluded to in a paper given by Whelan (1998) at a conference on Healthy Living Centres held in Gateshead in December 1998. Here, Whelan was describing the work of 'the Eldonians', a community regeneration programme based in Liverpool. The programme has achieved considerable success in replacing derelict land with new homes, care homes for the elderly, day nurseries for children and community centres in which a range of activities from shiatsu skills to reflexology and aromatherapy are used to overcome social isolation and increase levels of independence. Throughout the paper, Whelan placed great emphasis on using community action to overcome the culture of dependency. He suggests that 'it doesn't so much matter what the focus [of development] is, as *who determines it* because **that's** potentially the biggest health catalyst of all' and that 'action absolutely needs to be community led to **produce** any real change' (Whelan, 1998, p. 2, original emphasis).

In discussing future plans for the Eldonians, Whelan described the development of a major new, revolutionary, health/care profession – that of 'community therapeutic care'. This development recognised the skills based in the community that were available to address health issues and sought to formalise the role of people providing care in the community as well as simultaneously to attract further investment in these people to develop their skills and employment opportunities.

The developments described above arising from the work of Ward and McMahon (1998), the children's charities and the Eldonians highlight the emergence of a model of care grounded in everyday activities, embedded in families and the community, and drawing to a greater or lesser extent on established theories and knowledge bases. Each model is, however, being advocated because of identified deficiencies in existing models of professional practice that are considered to be too remote to engage directly in the problem, too episodic or too specialist and overprotective of the professional knowledge base to address the deeper problems associated with promoting holistic family health. The models suggested integrate existing professional practice, call on low-tech skills but recognise the expertise required to use them in complex family situations. They highlight acceptability to the family (for example, doing the ironing) as key to gaining access to and acceptance by the family. Finally, they recognise the importance of increasing the skill level of local people rather than importing skilled professionals from outside local communities as being a key feature for promoting family health in community settings.

The above discussion on the evolution of a new community care role mirrors some of the concerns expressed in a report produced by Manchester University (Steering Committee, 1996). The report found that, over the decade 1984–94, the growth rate for professionally qual-ified staff in nursing and midwifery was almost 1.5 times higher than that for support workers. As the report commented, it seemed to be that, since the introduction of supernumerary status for student nurses heralded in the UK by Project 2000, student labour had by and large been replaced by a qualified workforce. The report expressed surprise at this, suggesting that it was a professional rather than cost-effective management strategy.

The report made radical suggestions about the future health service workforce. It advocated the introduction of a 'generic carer' role. This role, which, according to the authors of the report, could be called 'nursing', would be the first-level training required by anyone wishing to pursue a career in the health service. This would include specialist nurses, doctors, physiotherapists, occupational therapists, speech and language therapists and even health service managers. The Steering Committee Report indicated neither the length of this training, the level of academic content nor the outcome. It did, however, suggest that this role could account for as much as 44 per cent of the current nursing workforce.

This idea is quite interesting as, at one level, it acknowledges the centrality of this generic role to all aspects of health care provision, to the extent that it recommends investing in training every health service employee in this role. However, as this role will only ever be a first-level training, for those who pursue it as a means of employment, their status and the status of this role in influencing health service policy will be undermined by the subsequent specialist and advanced training under-taken by all other health care professionals and managers.

While being seen as critical to care provision, the intellectual contribution that could be made to understanding issues of health promotion by a research-based approach to the generic role is clearly not recognised by the Steering Committee Report. Instead, it highlights the high burden of care that could be attended to by this workforce, which would free up the specialists to pursue the academic research necessary to develop the service. The report has clearly not moved beyond a definition of care-as-duty and implicitly accepts the custodial and containment elements associated with this type of provision as being adequate to meet the health care needs of the population being served.

The Steering Committee Report appears not to acknowledge the pivotal role that generic care could potentially play in transforming health in local communities and tackling health care needs that defy more traditional professional and specialist approaches to health care provision. In so doing, it fails to recognise the policy dilemmas described by Bulmer (1987) and Twigg (1989), outlined above. These dilemmas occur at the margins between formal and informal care, where the crucial role that generic care workers play in resolving these dilemmas through their everyday practice, and in so doing determining health or dependency at this margin, has yet to be fully explored.

In promoting health through communal action, the repeated message that comes through both academic and experiential accounts of this type of provision is the importance of engaging local communities in community development programmes. While individual members of a given community may occupy a formal provider role as a nurse, health service manager, consultant, social worker or residential care worker, they cannot speak or provide for the whole community through that role. Community development implies working at the boundaries between the formal and specialist service providers, and the informal domestic lives experienced by all members of society, regardless of their professional role.

Care-as-communal-action has sought to tackle the boundaries between different service providers and professional groups through such initiatives as HAZs and the Healthy Living Centres initiative. However, if the health care problems described in Vignettes 6 and 7 given earlier in this chapter are to be tackled effectively, more work needs to be undertaken in understanding the boundaries between care-as-communal-action and care-as-labour. The 'new roles' described above have recognised the limitations of existing forms of service provision and specialist professional practice. The type and level of skill required to work effectively at this boundary is only just beginning to be explored.

Caring for people with chronic illness

The topics raised by the three vignettes earlier in the chapter, and the above discussion of new and emerging roles and integrative practices, reflect many of the issues arising with regard to the long-term effective management of chronic illness and complex problems. Chapter 3 high-lighted the dominance of chronic illness in advanced industrial soci-eties. The work of Antonovsky (1996) and Lazarus (1992) suggests that the extent to which individuals and families will be able to live effec-tively with chronic illness will be in part determined by their previous access to the resources necessary to develop resilience and effective coping strategies. The adoption of a systems approach to studying health and illness illustrates the interrelationships between social struc-tures (resources, wealth, class and employment), the environment, communities and family and individual health. It enables an analysis of why individuals suffering from ostensibly the same physiological problem or disease may respond very differently to the disease process and therefore manifest different outcomes as a result of similar events (Burckhardt, 1987). In adopting a systems approach, it is, however, important to study the interactions that occur at the boundaries between the different systems. It is also necessary to recognise that the ability of individuals and families to cope effectively with illnesses is, in part, derived from their opportunities to access the resources located in other parts of the system.

Newby (1996) presents a conceptual framework for analysing the interaction of chronic illness with family and individual life cycles. She suggests that illness occurs within the context of an underlying order of the life course. The life course is characterised by known transitions, for example birth, adolescence, joining the labour market, marriage, parenthood and retirement. Individual and family development have in common the notion of phases marked by a constant change in building and maintaining roles and relationships through transitional periods of development. It is during periods of transition that the individual and the family are most vulnerable because previous individual and family life structures are reappraised in the light of new developmental tasks.

Newby suggests that the onset or exacerbation of illness in a family sets in motion a process of adaptation or socialisation to the illness. This process is prolonged in the case of chronic illness and can lead to a reappraisal of roles and responsibilities within the family. If the illness coincides with a period of natural transition in the family life cycle, it can alter a family's natural momentum, resulting in an increase in family stress. The ability of the individual or family to cope adequately with the increased stress may be in part determined by the level of resilience that they have been able to achieve.

Connelly (1987) highlights the importance of the concept of self-care in understanding the health care needs of chronically ill patients. Self-care is defined as the process whereby patients deliberately act on their own behalf in health promotion, the prevention of illness and the detection and treatment of health deviations. Connelly suggests that the chronically ill have special self-care needs because of the enduring nature of the illness and the way in which the illness and treatments tend to pervade all aspects of a person's lifestyle, including diet, mobility, exercise and energy level. Moreover, the treatment of chronic illness is usually on an ambulatory basis, that is, managed through appointments with specialists rather than as an in-patient. Patients are consequently the direct providers of their own care while the role of the professional changes to one of education, facilitator and supporter rather than direct provider. Moreover, many chronically ill people continue with their usual social roles and responsibilities, including remaining in employment and continuing to care for their families.

As Connelly highlights, chronically ill people need to incorporate the appropriate health/illness behaviours into the repertoire of their daily lives. She highlights the central role of nursing in facilitating this process. In particular, she identifies three main goals of nursing intervention in providing ambulatory care for chronically ill patients: (1) to stimulate and enhance effective self-care; (2) to reduce barriers to self-care; (3) to reinforce and support appropriate self-care by chronically ill patients.

Nolan and Grant (1989) highlight the conceptual similarities between self-care and health care: both intend to enhance health, prevent disease, evaluate symptoms and restore health. Consequently, they suggest, self-care forms a natural area of interest for the nursing profession with regard to both patients and their informal carers.

Gull (1987) reviews the adaptation of the chronically ill person to admission to hospital. She highlights how the disease management normally undertaken by the patient is interrupted by hospital personnel, some of whom take over self-care functions such as controlling medication.

Patients, however, rarely become totally passive. As Gull notes, knowledgeable patients frequently attempt to prevent staff members' errors, enter into the performance of technical procedures and provide some of their own continuity of care through the daily shift changes in staff. Gull points out that knowledgeable patients will frequently have their own way of managing the illness, which may not always conform to hospital practices, procedures and medical prescriptions. In managing chronic illness, the usual assumptions concerning the superiority of professional knowledge over the knowledge of the patient or recipient of the service may be unfounded and occasionally reversed. As Lazarus (1992) notes, hospitals are notoriously unresponsive to this aspect of patient management and can severely disrupt the integrity of the patient in the management of the illness.

Casey (1995) identifies the support of carers as being a crucial aspect of nursing. As a result of a survey of family involvement in the care of children in hospital, she identified four approaches adopted by nurses when communicating with parents. These included:

1. *communicating/nurse-centred: permission*, in which nurses adopted an authoritarian approach but assessed parents' wishes and allowed involvement on the nurses' terms;

2. *non-communication/nurse-centred: exclusion*, nurses excluding parents through numerous interpersonal practices, rules and regulations, not directly communicated by the nurses but learnt by the parents as a result of their experiences of interaction and observations of practice;

3. *non-communicating/person-centred: assumption*, where nurses made numerous ill-informed assumptions about the parents' ability to manage care and about the families' wishes and expectations. These opinions were subjective, unrecorded and not discussed with families;

4. *communicating/person-centred: negotiation*, there being some evidence that experienced older nurses are able to provide collaborative support for families in which decision making is based on a shared view of the problem. This was seen to involve a three-phase process beginning with eliciting requests and expectations, and followed by interaction, seeking consensus and finally decision making based on shared understanding.

Nolan and Grant (1989), in a review of the literature on informal care, contribute to an expanding body of knowledge that identifies support for informal carers as a key but frequently ignored aspect of nursing. Nolan and Grant acknowledge that, in advocating that nurses should address the needs of informal carers, it is important to recognise the organisational and ideological constraints that operate to undermine this activity. They suggest, however, that the onus rests with nursing as a profession to identify these constraints and actively work to overcome obstacles to supporting carers.

In looking at the needs of informal carers as depicted in the literature, Nolan and Grant identify the following factors as services that carers would like to receive: information on illness and treatment, the services available, choices and options, and the degree of flexibility with which services can be provided; skills training, especially in relation to nursing care, for example dealing with incontinence, lifting techniques and so on; emotional support, including being valued for the work that they were undertaking, receiving collegiate support in discussing the daily details of this work, and help with recognising and dealing with emotional responses to caring such as guilt, anger and hopelessness; setting the limits on their care and negotiating responsibilities with their dependant; and some form of regular respite from their role as carer. As a consequence of their own research, Nolan and Grant (1989) identified the need to develop a practice model of carer support to guide nurses in this activity. They advocated a stress-adaptation model within an educative-supportive framework.

Individualised patient care in nursing practice

Individualised patient care has been a prominent theme in the recent nursing literature. Initially arising from a recognition of the limitations of routinised and unresponsive approaches to care provision (Reed, 1992; May, 1995), it is accepted as enhancing caring by providing nursing in a more humane and therapeutic way (McMahon, 1991). Individualised care also acknowledges a change in understanding about the role and nature of being a patient. It builds on literature identifying that patients are not passive in their responses to disease processes or professional intervention, but actively contribute to the progression and resolution of problems arising from their health care needs.

May (1995), in a review of the development of individualised care in nursing, has identified a trend in which nursing moved from material or physical labour characterised by routines and tasks to an understanding of nursing that emphasises communication and relationships in order to reveal the patient's authentic character. This certainly reflects the work of Benner and Wrubel (1989) and the evolution of literature on caring in nursing (Kitson, 1999a, 1999b).

The movement from an emphasis on physical care to an emphasis on relationships has been subject to some criticism. Both Dunlop (1986) and Bjork (1995) express concern that, in moving into the realm of relationships, nurses are in danger of losing their professional identity and becoming indistinguishable from members of other occupations.

Bjork (1995) reviews literature illustrating the value that patients place on good physical care and technical skills in nursing. The close association demonstrated between physical care and routines in nursing has created a situation in which, in seeking to overcome routinised approaches to care, nursing has lost sight of a key aspect of its practice. At the same time, highlighting interpersonal relationships focuses on the role of the nurse as an individual in isolation from the collective environment in which nursing takes place. In a study designed to investigate factors that facilitate individualised care, Redfern (1996) has highlighted the importance of both the individual characteristics of the nurse and the organisation and resources available in the environment within which the nurse practises. Significantly, Redfern (1996) has also indicated the importance of patient characteristics in enabling individualised care to be achieved.

The personal qualities of nurses required to promote individualised patient care, as identified by Redfern, are a belief in individualised patient care, a passion for nursing, knowledge and experience, interpersonal skills and leadership qualities. These nursing characteristics, described by Redfern, clearly move beyond a conception of care-as-duty into a recognition of knowledgeable decision making and problem solving approaches to nursing associated with care-as-ethical-position.

The organisational characteristics identified by Redfern to promote individualised patient care include ward organisation that must ensure continuity for patients, provide support for students/trained staff and involve qualified staff in direct patient care. Redfern's findings reinforce the importance of retaining care-as-labour as a central focus of nursing activity by all grades of staff. The organisation of staffing, roles and workload must ensure 'adequate' staffing levels and an appropriate skill mix; good administrative support through ward clerks is also vital. The sister's role in supporting, supervising, encouraging, role modelling, leadership and the management of individualised patient care is also essential. Support for her from her managers is also required. There must also be commitment to individualised patient care from all members of the multidisciplinary team, enabling decisions to be taken by the most appropriate staff member in relation to the underlying problem.

The characteristic of the patient that will promote individualised care is a propensity for partnership in the care process, as for example with longer-stay, younger, higher-dependency patients. From the patient's perspective, Redfern's work indicates that short, crisis-orientated, episodic encounters with services are not conducive to understanding or resolving the complex problems encountered by many people when striving to achieve health. Such short encounters with services reduce the effectiveness of nurses and other professionals in addressing these problems through individualised patient care.

It is possible to conjecture that the difficulties hospitals face in dealing with complex problems such as those presented in Vignettes 6 and 7 arise from their overemphasis on physiological care and their failure to address the psychosocial dimensions of care. In such circumstances, the role of hospitals in meeting the needs of patients with complex problems is marginal, and the technical interventions provided costly but largely ineffective.

A lack of co-ordination is frequently given as a reason why services fail to address complex needs. It is frequently assumed that this can be resolved by the development of multiprofessional teams. Øvretveit (1993) argues strongly for the need to set up managed teams in situations where spontaneous networks have not developed. He claims that much can be achieved by paying attention to the co-ordination of structures, resources and staff. Øvretveit proposes that managed teams frequently fail because members are divided between the team and their own profession in relation to their loyalty, membership, management and geographical location. Also identified are a lack of formal authority for team procedures, priority setting, review and negotiation with purchasers of legitimate areas of team activity.

According to Øvretveit (1993), successful multiprofessional teams require a reconfiguration of traditional organisational structures in order to create new staff groupings reflecting changing priorities. Care-as-ethical-position is about particularising the integration of diverse service provision to meet the specific needs of a given individual or family. At the same time, it addresses a holistic approach to problem solving by integrating the biopsychosocial dimensions of the situation into an analysis of the problem in order to arrive at a solution. This means that individuals with ostensibly the same problem at a physical level may require very different forms of service input to accommodate the psychosocial dimensions of the problem.

In redesigning care streams through reconfiguring multiprofessional teams, there is clearly a need to identify the ethical and theoretical framework within which care is being delivered. This is required in order to develop a rationale for the particular configuration of the team and to prevent a new but equally abstract set of assumptions about need to dominate provision and obscure problem resolution at an individual level.

In reflecting on the theoretical development of individualised care in nursing, May (1995) raises a number of questions about the ideas that underpin the 'invention' of this type of care. In particular, he is concerned about the gradual conflation of individualised care and of individualism in nursing's rhetoric about the patient. He asks:

> What if the patient does not see him/herself as an active collaborative, partner in care, or as an expert in his/her own health, or fails to see the realm of psychosocial as one into which the nurse is legitimately entitled to intrude? Such a patient may actively resist [participation]... and is easily categorised as non-compliant and maladaptive. (May, 1995, p. 86)

The notion of intrusion goes to the heart of developing individualised care in nursing. The concept of individualised care allows for a differentiated approach to care based on clinical nursing judgement. To impose intrusive care on all patients irrespective of a health needs analysis reintroduces routinised approaches to nursing, albeit designed to address individual need. A key aspect of skilled nursing in individualised care appears to be the ability to distinguish between those patients and carers experiencing unresolved and enduring health care needs, who would benefit from a more 'intrusive' partnership approach to nursing, and those patients and carers who are able to address these needs for themselves independently of the health care system.

Northway (1997), in discussing the needs of disabled people as described in the disability literature, highlights how, for many disabled people, professionals including nurses are increasingly being viewed as part of their experience of oppression. Intrusive, individualised care could be construed as furthering rather than relieving the experience of oppression on the part of disabled people. However, as Northway points out, oppression can arise from well-intentioned acts and can be passive as well as active. Doing nothing for fear of being intrusive is not anti-oppressive: it merely reinforces the dominance of technological medicine as Vignettes 6 and 7 illustrate, giving rise to increasing isolation for people suffering from disabilities. Northway suggests that nursing as a profession has the choice of either running the risk of being seen increasingly as part of the problem of disability, or seeking to work in partnership with disabled people to become part of the solution by adopting anti-oppressive practices. Part of this necessarily involves seeing the disabled person as an ordinary individual with a disability rather than focusing primarily on the needs arising from the disability.

Conclusion

This chapter has described the development of nursing within a multi-professional, multi-agency context. It has illustrated the centrality of individualised care to resolving many of the most pressing problems confronting the resolution of health care needs within families. New ways of practising have been explored, and the pivotal role of nursing in addressing issues arising at the interface between formal and informal care has been described.

It would appear that nursing cannot escape the conundrum described by May (1995). To return to traditional nursing practices based on routinised and undifferentiated approaches to nursing provision reinforces oppression and isolation for patients with complex and enduring health care needs. Having recognised the limitations of this approach to nursing and having embarked on a journey to resolve this problem, nursing must continue to work to identify how to establish collaborative and effective partnerships with patients and their carers.

The pivotal and central role of nursing in working at the boundaries of formal and informal care is increasingly being acknowledged (Kitson, 1987; Nolan and Grant, 1989; Casey, 1995). The close association between nursing work and caring work performed by family members, as described in Chapter 4, means that nursing may benefit from research into how people organise women's work in the community. Studies of this type of work may provide prototypes for models of how to organise nursing in health service settings.

In suggesting this, it is recognised that nursing is different in its function from other health care professions. This difference does not necessarily equate with less importance in its impact on patient outcome and cost-effectiveness in health care. What it does mean is that it may not conform to traditional assumptions about professionalisation, management, hierarchy and accountability structures, nor does it necessarily produce outcomes that can be measured according to normative criteria. This does not give rise to the need to be complacent and dismissive, but instead suggests the need to investigate nursing and ways of working in nursing that are conducive to its function and will give rise to more appropriate conceptualisations of outcomes. The next chapter reviews skill mix and workload in nursing, while the final chapter addresses issues of accountability and the daily organisation of nursing care in hospital and community settings.

Chapter 7

Measuring Nursing – Progress and Pitfalls

The previous chapter highlighted a growing awareness of the problems of delivering services that interface with informal family care. Nursing's public responsibility for care as labour provides an entrée into family care and the possibility of studying this complex area of public service provision through the practice experiences of nurses delivering care at this interface. Graham (1984) highlighted the moral distinction experienced by families between contacting services in response to physical symptoms and for preventative health care such as vaccinations and dental care, and contacting services because of difficulty coping with the stresses and strains of family care. To do the former is considered good care by the family and bestows moral worth on family members. To do the latter suggests a failure on the part of the family and invites adverse moral judgement. May's (1995) critique of individualised care in nursing, discussed at the end of the previous chapter, highlights the sensitivities surrounding suggestions that nurses should intrude into the personal arena of individual and family coping strategies.

Care as labour is of necessity intimate care. In practice, it includes helping patients with a full range of personal tending activities, including urinary and faecal elimination, personal hygiene, feeding, skin integrity, appearance and sexual functioning. There is a substantial literature in nursing that points to the use of routines (Menzies, 1960; Procter, 1989a; Lawler, 1991) both as a way of setting the boundaries on legitimate nursing work and as a way of managing the intimate and invasive aspects of nursing care. This chapter reviews this literature and discusses the centrality of nursing routines as a method of providing 24-hour care, which cannot be given by a single individual and, therefore, requires a collective approach to care provision.

The chapter begins, however, with a review of the literature on measuring nursing workload and skill mix in nursing. The chapter argues that, by concentrating on measuring tasks to be performed arising from physical disability or dependency, workload measurement in nursing perpetuates an approach to care that conforms to Kitson's (1993) description of care-as-duty, as non-individualised and potentially oppressive.

Measuring nursing workload

'Expenditure on nursing in the Hospital and Community Health Services of England and Wales was almost £5 billion in 1988–89. This was 36% of health authorities' revenue expenditure and almost half of their salary bill' (Audit Commission, 1991, p. 3). The NHS employs over 332,000 nurses, midwives and health visitors (DoH, 1999). Nurses number close to five million in the 50 countries of the WHO European Region, ranging from just over 25 per 10,000 population in Hungary to just over 135 per 10,000 population in Norway in the early 1990s (Salvage and Heijnen, 1997). In numerical terms alone, nursing clearly represents a considerable force within health care.

Despite the large number of nurses employed by the health service and the considerable sum of public money expended on their salaries and on the education, development and management of nurses, very little progress appears to have made in providing a coherent framework for answering the question 'How many nurses do we need?' in a given ward, department, hospital, specialism or community unit, or indeed in the NHS itself.

In recognition of this problem, numerous formulae have been developed to help managers to identify appropriate staffing levels on wards and, more recently, in community units. Nurses themselves, however, continue to feel underresourced and overstretched in attempting to meet the nursing care needs of patients. This frequently leads to friction between nurses and their managers and a feeling of failure in reaching a consensus that identifies the level of nursing resources appropriate to a given area.

The lack of progress in achieving a consensus on appropriate levels of nurse staffing and skill mix cannot be attributed to a lack of research or a failure to invest resources in considering these questions. Instead, these questions have dominated the Department of Health (DoH) agenda for nursing research since the inception of the NHS itself, if not before. The DoH has systematically reviewed this research over the past

15 years. As a result, a number of reports have been produced detailing and summarising the findings from this research (DHSS, 1982a, 1982b, 1983). More recently, Hurst (1993) has undertaken a comprehensive review of this literature covering more than 80 separate studies designed to develop techniques for managing nursing resources.

A substantial number of different formulae for measuring nursing work have been produced. They have in common, as the work of Hurst (1993) illustrates, a predominant methodology, one derived from operational research and utilising variations on the theme of activity analysis. Activity analysis is a method whereby non-participant observations of nursing work are undertaken and the average amount of time that nurses spend on subunits of nursing work, such as taking a blood pressure or giving out medication, is calculated. The calculations are adjusted for factors identified as affecting nursing workload, such as patient dependency, administrative support, ancillary support, the size of the ward and bed occupancy. Other factors, for example, sickness and absence levels, meal and tea breaks, annual leave and other 'time-out' factors, may also be included in the formula.

Once the average timings for nursing activities have been derived and the weighting attributable to the factors affecting the delivery of nursing care has been identified, a formula for measuring nursing workload is produced. Further observation, using the formula, is undertaken. This is used to calculate the amount of nursing time required to meet the workload generated by the service.

Carr-Hill and Jenkins-Clarke (1995, p. 222) suggest that 'Ideally, activity analysis should be undertaken on each ward, day and night, for a given time period and repeated at intervals in order that the parameter reliably reflects changes in the pattern of ward activity.' They acknowledge, however, the difficulties in doing this and suggest it that it is 'not surprising' that managers frequently import timings from other parts of the hospital, other sites and the company supplying the system.

There are two major problems with activity analysis discussed in this chapter. The first is the tautology implicit in activity analysis, which produces measurements of nursing work, assumed to be objective because they are quantified, but which fail to link nursing activities to patient outcomes. The second is the definition of nursing work produced by activity analysis, which focuses on activities that can be discretely measured. In so doing, it renders invisible the integration of activities frequently achieved by nurses, as well as all aspects of nursing such as problem solving and ethical decision making that cannot be delineated as discrete tasks.

Nursing workload: lack of progress

The current emphasis in health care on producing costed packages of care for distinct patient groups, (i) to identify the level of resourcing required by the patient group as a basis for funding; (ii) to compare costs between health care providers; and (iii) to compare the costs and effectiveness of different treatment modalities, represents perhaps the single most important research agenda within the current research and development strategy in the NHS. Given the cost of nursing to the NHS, nursing has not been exempt from this agenda.

What, perhaps, distinguishes nursing is that it has been researching this agenda for considerably longer than any other professional group. Early studies can be traced back to the work of Goddard (1953) and Barr (1967), both of whom undertook research utilising activity analysis as a basis for measuring the amount of nursing care received by patients. More recent studies have produced more sophisticated formulae but have adopted very similar methodological techniques.

In a comparative study of these systems, Jenkins-Clarke (1992) contrasted three different approaches to measuring nursing workload:

1. Dependency-driven approaches, that is, systems producing workload requirements based mainly on measuring the dependency of ward patients on nursing care usually related to the performance of basic activities of daily living. Examples used in the study were Criteria for Care and the South-East Nursing System, or SENS.

2. Task-orientated approaches, that is, systems relying on recording and predicting nursing interventions for individual patients. The Financial Information Project (FIP) was the example used in the study.

3. Care plan-driven approaches, that is, systems measuring workload by producing nursing care plans that are then used to predict the workload. Exelcare is a computerised care plan-orientated system used in the study.

Carr-Hill and Jenkins-Clarke (1995) used each of the above nursing management workload systems to calculate the nurse staffing requirement on three wards over six days ($n = 18$ days of data collected). In addition, data were collected on shift patterns on the wards, the proportion of untrained staff, the case mix groupings of patients, and nursing outcome. Their results demonstrated a difference in staffing costs of £68,006 per annum per ward, depending on which system was used. A quite high correlation between the estimates of over/understaffing produced by each system and the per capita hours worked was found, but no obvious pattern could be detected to explain this. Quality, measured by nursing outcome, varied inversely with overstaffing – that is, more staff did not equate with meeting more nursing outcomes – but correlated weakly with skill mix. In other words, overstaffing, as measured by these systems, using untrained staff does not lead to a corresponding increase in quality.

In commenting on these differences, Carr-Hill and Jenkins-Clarke (1995) urge caution about 'the over-ambitious claims made for many measurement systems' (p. 224) and suggest that nursing workload management systems must be tested for practicability, reliability and validity before being promoted or adopted on a large scale. They also recognise the political context of management in health care and acknowledge that nursing workload measurement systems, along with other attempts to produce empirical measures of NHS activity and effectiveness, tend to become distorted by managerial agendas and market forces.

The findings of Carr-Hill and Jenkins-Clarke (1995) are reinforced in a review by the Audit Commission (1991) of data currently collected on nurse staffing levels. The Audit Commission found a large variation between districts in both the average number of qualified nurses per patient day and the proportion of qualified staff employed on acute wards. The Audit Commission found, however, that the lack of a commonly accepted measure of patient dependency or nursing workload prevented a more detailed analysis. They recognised that comparative data on the staffing of outwardly similar wards across the country can provoke questions of equity in care provision. They recognised, however, that local factors and differences in the quality of care provided on wards with differing levels and mixes of staffing and availability of support services must be taken into consideration when reviewing ward staffing before useful conclusions can be drawn about potential efficiency improvements.

It seems that, despite the extensive amount of research already undertaken into nurse staffing levels and skill mix, very little progress has been made towards answering the question 'How many nurses do we need?' These systems may help managers at a local level in the day-to-day distribution of existing nursing resources within a given unit or hospital. They seem unable, however, to address issues of equity in the distribution of nursing resources between units, hospitals and geographical districts, as wide and seemingly inexplicable variations continue. Moreover, if, as suggested by Carr-Hill and Jenkins-Clarke (1995), it is necessary to undertake a detailed activity analysis in every clinical area in which these systems are to be used (not to mention repeated activity analysis to capture any change in timings brought about by a change in throughput and practice as services develop), the effectiveness of these tools must be considered.

The frustration that both nurses at ward level and their managers feel in relation to setting and maintaining the nurse staffing level appears to be justified. At the end of the day, these systems seem consistently to throw the onus back onto local managers to determine an appropriate staffing level within local contexts. It is possible to suggest that the utilisation of these systems represents a considerable cost to the NHS, and the cost–benefit of these systems must also be evaluated, particularly in the light of their failure to produce valid and reliable information.

Activity analysis: a tautological approach to measuring workload in nursing

In a review published as long ago as 1982, Gault, a lecturer in operational research in University College Galway and a post-graduate researcher in the Health Services Operational research unit at the University of Strathclyde, Glasgow, undertook a detailed critique of the Aberdeen formula, an early nursing workload system that was the genesis for many of the systems in use today. As well as highlighting a number of technical problems with the Aberdeen formula, Gault highlighted three major philosophical problems with workload measurement in nursing that he felt were applicable to any system that was based on some form of activity analysis:

- The first was a belief – Gault actually used the word 'faith' – in the scientific method as a means of determining nursing requirement.
- The second was the mechanistic view of nursing that this gave rise to.
- The third was a belief in expertise.

In discussing the problem of the faith in scientific method, Gault cites Norwich and Senior, who in 1971 asked:

> how is the nurse allocator to know how many nurses are really required in the absence of any way of measuring the workload generated by patients?

Subjective measures, followed by the arbitrary decision of senior nurses are not satisfactory'. (Norwich and Senior, 1971, p. 17)

Science was seen to offer a non-subjective (objective) means of reaching non-arbitrary (that is, rational) decisions. The use of the scientific method as depicted in the Aberdeen formula was seen to provide a 'reliable means of predicting the need of patients, measuring the performance of nurses and then matching the two to yield the number of nurses required' (Gault, 1982, p. 69).

A major problem with this approach to measuring nursing workload is that the categories used to classify nursing, and the subsequent costings of nursing time calculated from these categories, are derived from historical patterns of nurse staffing. If, for example, certain wards have historically been better staffed, the particular way in which nurses use the additional resources to provide care will be measured in the activity analysis. Such an approach merely serves to capture historical diversity in the distribution of nursing resources and formalise this diversity in an authoritative workload indicator. It does not establish the appropriateness of the activities performed in terms of their impact on patient care or the resolution of patient's nursing needs.

Most studies recognise this problem and attempt to build in some quality control measure. This measure is, however, invariably based on expert opinion, activities being reviewed by expert panels (as in Aberdeen) or more recently by the nurses themselves to assess the appropriateness of the activities being measured to the needs of the patient. This approach to quality control recognises nursing competence as it is based wholly on professional judgement and, therefore, reinforces professional aspirations in nursing. It fails, however, to challenge nursing practice to substantiate the claims about good care made in these studies, or even to demonstrate an effective organisation of provision. Nursing workload formulae are, therefore, based on professional judgement and cannot claim to be evidence based.

The processes involved in quantifying nursing workload are insufficient on their own to produce an objective measure of nursing workload. Objectivity requires more than the simple process of quantification. Studies to date designed to measure nurse workload have simply provided a numerical description of that workload. The complexity of nursing has demanded an increasing level of sophistication in the production of these systems, but focusing on the production of increasingly sophisticated systems has served to obscure their essentially descriptive nature.

Throughout the history of the development of these systems, nursing workload has continued to be defined as what nurses say it is or, more empirically, what nurses do. Consequently, these tools are tautological in that the definition of nursing work inherent in them is derived from empirical observations of nursing practice. Nursing practice has itself been shaped by historical approaches to setting the nursing budget, by the local availability of qualified nurses and by prevailing patterns of skill mix. At no point in history has either the level or skill mix provided in nursing been acknowledged as being adequate by all parties, particularly if the distribution of nurses across specialities and geographical locations is taken into account.

Nursing workload management systems fail, therefore, to provide nurses with the key data required to resolve ongoing disputes. Instead, such systems assume that current arrangements for organising the provision of nursing care are in fact optimal and this is what is measured. The ongoing debates about nurse staffing level arise from a failure either to provide adequate staffing to meet currently defined optimal levels of provision, or more usually to agree what is an optimal standard of provision within the hospital or provider unit. The failure in many hospitals to reach an agreement between general managers, nursing managers and clinical nurses over what is an optimal level of nursing care within the hospital exposes perhaps the biggest weakness of these studies. By failing to demonstrate the effectiveness of nursing care in terms of patient outcome, nurses are left with tools that only quantify workload. But, workload on its own, no matter how worthy, is insufficient to command resources in the cost-conscious political climate of the NHS. This leaves nurses vulnerable to continued pressure to reduce the staffing level or alter skill mix in order to contain the budget.

Management tools that base measurements of workload on the prevailing patterns of provision and distribution of nursing resources, as measured during activity analysis, will always be questioned by those who dispute the adequacy of existing service provision (RCN, 1992, 1993) or consider it excessive (Steering Committee, 1996). Quantifying the problem merely provides data on which to base the debate, but it can never provide evidence for resolving the debate. Evidence to settle the debate requires a more experimental, less descriptive approach to the development of nurse management information systems. Surprisingly, despite the large number of studies that have been undertaken, many of which were commissioned by the DoH with very respectable research budgets, few experimental studies have been conducted in relation to skill mix and nurse staffing levels.

Methodological confusion

There has been a tendency in nursing research to align quantification with positivist (cause and effect) approaches to research and with experimentation, as well as to assume that descriptive, non-experimental research is confined to qualitative methodologies. The arena of research into nursing workload demonstrates problems with this assumption. It is equally possible to produce quantitative research that is highly descriptive, subjective and non-experimental but which produces large amounts of statistical data that lull the reader into the sense that this amount of statistical information must be positivist in orientation and, therefore, objective. Similarly, theoretical critiques of this approach that use qualitative methods are dismissed as being anecdotal and subjective. The stage is set for the continual repetition of methodological errors because of a failure to address the more deep-rooted theoretical and methodological issues.

The issue of methodological confusion is the substance of the second criticism of nursing workload measurement systems made by Gault (1982), who identifies the mechanistic view of nursing implicit in the methodologies used in these systems. He suggests that these methods assume that each workload element measured is determined by a characteristic of the patient; that is, workload is regarded as the outcome of a cause-and-effect process in which the patient caused the effect – nursing. This is the point at which the predictive quality assumed by these systems is located. By identifying and quantifying patient needs (cause), it is possible to predict nursing workload (effect).

Gault dismisses this conceptualisation of nursing as decidedly ill informed, suggesting that nurses have much more control over their workload than this mechanistic equation implies. Nurses can and do make choices about how they spend their time, and these choices may not conform to the timings captured in the activity analysis, hence the findings of Carr-Hill and Jenkins-Clarke (1995) that the timings lack reliability and are non-transferable, arguably because nurses are fully aware of patient needs and adjust the way in which these needs are met according to the local context of service provision.

The problem of reliability found to pervade the use of nurse workload measurement systems relates directly back to the description of nursing given in Chapter 5 as managing the 24-hour life space of the patient. In that chapter, it was suggested that nursing is about managing the personal needs of patients and the impact of their health crisis on the organisation of their daily activities. At the same time, nurses seek to integrate the complex demands arising from the patients' personal situation with the smooth running of the health service in order to schedule provision and maximise efficient use of expensive resources. It follows that nurses do this not only in relation to the totality of health service provision, but also in relation to the supply of their own labour.

Fundamental to nursing, therefore, is skill at managing the needs of patients within the local context of service provision and within the level of nursing resources and skills currently available on the ward. It is arguably the consequences of this highly skilled management that are measured so carefully and in so much detail by operational researchers. The difficulties with reliability arise because nurses fine-tune their activity in response to changes in patient needs and the service capacity to meet these needs.

This definition of what nurses do indicates that nursing is not about providing a direct treatment modality, as perhaps other professions do, and it is this that renders nursing invisible in a system that is increasingly about productivity. The health service is currently collecting large quantities of data on operational performance, including such things as how many operations are performed, how many treatment sessions are undertaken by physiotherapists and occupational therapists, how many drugs are prescribed and by whom.

The problem confronting the nursing service is that the tools that have traditionally been used to measure the contribution of nursing have assumed that nursing, like other health care professions, is about treatment. Nursing workload systems have, therefore, striven to count the number of treatments provided by nurses, and they have done this by counting the number of tasks that nurses perform and equating tasks with treatments. Treatments are, after all, the primary purpose of the NHS, and it would be demeaning to nursing not to acknowledge its role in this. The conflation of tasks with treatments in nursing is both confusing and unhelpful. As the work of Carr-Hill and Jenkins-Clarke (1995) and Hurst (1993) illustrates, it amounts to adding up all the tasks undertaken by nurses to identify the nursing contribution and then providing neatly costed nursing packages.

It is possible to argue that the more nursing tries to conform to the planned and costed nursing activities identified by these systems as being appropriate to the needs of the patient, the more it fails to be able to respond to the divergent needs of the patient and the health service organisation, and to work to bring them into some sort of harmony. What is interesting is that, while equating nursing tasks with treatments on the one hand, nursing tasks have not been subject to the same level of systematic evaluation associated with the introduction of new treatments or technologies. Perhaps because many of these tasks are derived from the work of other professionals, it is assumed that their effectiveness has been fully evaluated before delegation. Consequently nursing workload management systems record fluid balance chart timed at one minute (Hurst, 1993) without questioning the purpose of the fluid balance chart in the first instance, taking this to be either self-evident or previously evaluated by the delegating professional.

Taken together, the two criticisms of Gault (1982) give rise to his third concern, a belief in expertise. Here, Gault suggests that health service managers, be they nurses or non-nurses, have listened more to and placed greater value on the technical advice of experts, usually operational researchers, to solve management problems and dilemmas, than that of the nurses themselves. While these experts could and have produced numerous expert systems, as demanded of them, they cannot be expected to address deeper fundamental questions concerning the development of nursing for a specific patient group or health care problem: only nurses can identify the contribution that they can or could make to patient outcomes, and managers decide its value.

Nursing workload: the way forward

In contrast to the vast volumes of descriptive data produced by nursing workload management systems, it would seem that a better starting point would be some sort of succinct encompassing definition of nursing. Chapter 5 provided a description of nursing as a responsive profession, a profession that provides round-the-clock care in order to manage the '24-hour life space of the patient', to ensure that the patient is in the right place at the right time in the right condition – physically, mentally, emotionally and socially – in order to be receptive to and able to benefit from the therapeutic health care inputs of other professionals.

This description of nursing is mirrored in the Audit Commission's report (1991). The report suggests that the central focus of nursing is managing a group of patients and organising the support services. This involves working in a team with other nurses, doctors, paramedics and social workers, as well as assessing, planning, implementing, teaching and co-ordinating, monitoring, reviewing and advising on different aspects of the care process. The Audit Commission goes on to emphasise the nurses' role in co-ordinating care of the whole patient through devolved management, an expanding clinical role and support tasks.

It is possible to argue that nursing, like other aspects of health care, is characterised by a seemingly infinite demand for resources. No matter how many nurses are supplied, there will never be quite enough to meet the demand for nursing care. Nursing research has increasingly demonstrated the potential range and depth of patient problems encountered by nurses. Both James (1992) and Smith (1992) have described the emotional labour performed by nurses as part of their everyday nursing activities. Recognising this work and acknowledging it as a legitimate nursing activity uncovers a potentially huge level of demand from patients for emotional and psychological support, as evidenced by the vignettes provided in Chapter 6.

Early work by Menzies (1960) highlighted how the organisation of nursing work into tasks and functional activities distanced nurses from confronting and engaging with the full emotional and psychological consequences for patients of the onset or progression of their illness. Work was instead allocated to nurses as a series of tasks that were performed on all the patients who required those tasks during that shift. Nurses worked with each of the patients on a specific task and then moved on to the next patient. Nursing workload was contained and delineated by the tasks to be completed. Once the tasks had been completed, nurses could assume that their work was done. This approach to nursing care was described as both routinised and ritualistic as it responded to patients not as individuals but as diseased bodies that required certain tasks to be completed for health to be sustained and recovery aided.

More recently, Alaszweski (1977) and Procter (1989a) have demonstrated how the development of nursing work routines in hospitals sets the parameters on workload in the absence of any other way of determining when the work is complete. While nurses may not have the resources or skills to meet all of the manifest needs of patients, they have at least completed the ward routine and can go off duty with a certain feeling of satisfaction at a good day's work well done. Without the ward routine, nurses would always be at the mercy of unmet need, and no matter how hard they worked or how great their achievements, they would never feel any sense of satisfaction with their work as all they would be aware of would be what they failed to achieve. Nurses' accomplishments would go unnoticed by everyone, including themselves.

Lawler (1991) highlights the use of routines as a way of managing the intimate aspects of nursing work. Much of nursing activity involves bearing witness to or facilitating activities that are normally undertaken in private, such as urinary and faecal elimination, personal hygiene and care of the appearance. Alternatively, patients may need assistance with activities that assume independence, such as feeding, drinking and dressing. Lawler describes how nurses use routines as a structured way of invading patient privacy. The intimate activity witnessed or performed on a stranger, while highly irregular if undertaken outside a health care environment, is regulated by the routine and rendered acceptable and unquestioned. The inappropriate performance of the routine on the wrong patient or in the wrong setting is, however, an error and an irregularity that breaks social taboos in the same way as performing the activity outside a health care setting. Routines, therefore, facilitate intimate care and demarcate the provision of this care, enabling nursing work to be performed.

In conjunction with routines, Lawler (1991) also describes how nurses perform their tasks unobtrusively. They might be witnessing a highly personal act such as a patient of the opposite sex passing urine, but the conversation will be unobtrusive, about a television programme they have watched or concerning the cards received by the patient. According to Lawler, this strategy is used by nurses to indicate that they find the potentially embarrassing situation normal and uninteresting. Lawler suggests that it is these techniques which enable nurses to provide intimate care without embarrassing either patients or themselves. According to Lawler, nurses will only discuss the intimate activity if there is a problem and then in such a way as to make witnessing the problem a normal, ordinary, everyday event for the nurse, one not worthy of special comment. Unobtrusive approaches to nursing render intimate nursing care activities normal for the nurse, making them bearable for the patient.

May (1995), in his critique of the adoption of individualised approaches to care in nursing, recognises a tension between the nurse's authority to organise care and a fundamental concern in nursing to promote patient autonomy. He suggests that tension may exist between what patients want or desire and what nurses are able to provide, promoting patient autonomy undermines the authority vested in nurses to manage care.

In this context, Graham's analysis of the routines embodied in family care appears to be relevant. Graham (1984) suggests that routines pattern the day. Tensions, such as those described by May (1995), and the competing demands on the carer that they evoke, are managed by reference to the routine. Special requests will be met if time, resources and the carer permit. The routine enables nurses to convey to patients the collective demands of all patients and the right of nurses to prioritise their care to ensure that it is distributed appropriately between the competing needs of different patients.

MacGuire (1988), in discussing the nursing care needs of elderly people, suggests that dependency of all kinds – interpersonal, organisational and structural – must be of interest to nurses. She describes how the notion of dependency is inextricably linked to infancy and childhood: a state of being totally reliant on another person for everything. With children, MacGuire suggests, the natural process of maturation serves to counterbalance any tendency that the parent may have to keep the child dependent. In nursing, particularly of the elderly, no such counterbalancing process exists. In nursing the elderly, the needs of the carer and the patient converge in a way that might create increasing dependence on the part of the elderly person unless a very strong counterbalance to dependency is put in place. MacGuire suggests that the implicit model found in nursing usually turns out to be one that creates dependency.

Northway (1997) discusses how dignity is maintained for disabled people by recognising and addressing their individual integrity rather than attending just to the physical needs arising from their disability. Routinised unobtrusive nursing is essential for accomplishing tasks of an intimate nature, but practice needs to recognise the integrity of the individual in receipt of the care if it is not to become oppressive for the patient and damaging for the nurse.

It follows that routines are a powerful force in nursing work and should not be dismissed lightly. Nursing research has, however, tended to focus on the negative aspects of nursing routines, highlighting their dehumanising effect on patients and nurses alike (Menzies, 1960; Baker, 1983). The development of academic nursing and the professional aspirations of nursing have also contributed to a desire to promote patient-centred, individualised care, which for want of a better definition is, as May (1995) suggests, frequently assumed to be contrary to the provision of care mediated by routines.

This has resulted in a change in the organisation and provision of nursing care. The introduction of both primary nursing (Manthey, 1980) and team nursing was designed to increase nurse–patient continuity and facilitate the development of a therapeutic relationship between the nurse and the patient. Developments in nursing theory and nursing models (McKenna, 1997), the introduction of the nursing process (Kratz, 1979) and primary nursing (Pearson, 1988), while constructive professional responses to the shortcomings identified by nurse researchers such as Menzies (1960) and Baker (1983), have strug-

gled to provide alternative structures for setting boundaries on legitimate nursing concerns.

Part of the problem, as May (1995) acknowledges, is the conflation
of individualised care with individualism in nursing. In other words,
the collective activity that characterises the practice of nursing in
providing 24-hour care to a group of patients has been lost and replaced
by an exclusive emphasis on one-to-one nurse–patient relationships. As
a result of this emphasis, nurses are exposed to an increasing insight
into the problems and anxieties experienced by the patient and family
or informal carers. Nursing theories and models developed to help
nurses to address these problems reflect individualistic definitions of
health. Consequently, they do not provide a framework for helping
nurses to distinguish between and prioritise the competing needs of
different patients for their time and attention.

It seems that the more knowledge that nursing develops, the more
needs it uncovers. In turn, the more needs that are uncovered, the more
difficult it becomes to develop workload tools that provide an afford-
able level of nursing provision. The discussion of nurse workload
management systems earlier in this chapter highlighted how, by
depending on activity analysis, these systems assumed that nursing care
was a static measurable entity. The discussion of routines in this section
indicates that, rather than measuring patients' needs for nursing care,
these systems simply measure nursing routines.

Given the problems of setting boundaries on nursing work, other
than through routines, it follows that identifying the number of nurses
required and the skill mix needed will always be relative to nurses'
understanding of patient needs and the capacity of the organisation to
respond effectively to these needs. Nurses will assess the capacity of the
staff available on a given shift to cover the range of nursing care needs of
the patients. The routine will mediate between competing patient
needs and afford nurses some degree of flexibility in managing care.

MacGuire (1988) has recognised the interaction between nursing
activities and the promotion of either self-care or dependency. She has
highlighted the value of measuring dependency, not as a basis for
measuring workload, which assumes that patient dependency is independent of nursing activities, but as a means of measuring outcome in
nursing practice. Here, dependency is used to measure the outcome of
nursing practices that aim to promote self-care and independence,
which are central to much nursing theory.

However, as MacGuire cautions, the routine may, without an
explicit nursing model, implicitly promote dependency. Some nurses

will recognise this and may bring this problem to the attention of management. The extent to which care can be changed to adopt a model that promotes self-care will, however, largely depend on the skill mix and number of nurses available and the stability of and resources available in the care environment. Nursing workload management systems have failed to capture the dynamic quality that exists between the level of skill and resource available to nurses and the capacity of nurses to provide care that promotes health rather than maintains dependency.

There has been considerable theoretical development in nursing, giving rise to numerous nursing models that are advocated as a basis for practice. Most of the models, and indeed the theories from which they derive, are academic constructs; very few have evolved from practice. Consequently, the gap between theory development and practice in nursing remains wide. The following overview of nursing models illustrates this divide and highlights some of the difficulties associated with transferring these theoretical models into practice. The remainder of this chapter illustrates how nursing theory could, potentially, be used to test the effects on patients of using different levels of staffing and skill mix.

Using nursing theories and models to identify nurse staffing levels and skill mix

Fawcett (1989) suggests that it is possible to divide nursing models into two categories, reflecting two major differences in philosophical beliefs or 'world views' about person–environment interrelationships.

One world view focuses on change in person–environment interrelationships and is derived from notions of humanistic psychology that emphasise growth and development. Within this world view, change and growth are continual and desirable, progress is valued and realisation of one's potential is emphasised.

The other world view focuses not on change but on persistence and stability – the maintenance of patterns over time. This world view maintains that stability is natural and normal, that persistence is endurance in time and is produced by a synthesis of growth and stability. The persistence world view emphasises equilibrium and balance.

Both of these world views can be linked back to definitions of health presented in Chapter 2. Concepts of personal growth and the realisation of potential are implicit within many universal theories of health and health promotion, while concepts of balance, stability and

Caring for Health

Table 7.1   Comparison of the nature of nursing in five nursing
models classified within the change-as-stability paradigm

Nursing model	Nature of nursing
Roy (1984)	Manipulation of stimuli to foster coping
Orem (1991)	Systems that address self-care requisites
King (Frey, 1995)	Goal-orientated interaction
Johnson (1980)	External force towards balance
Neuman (Reed, 1993)	Stress-reducing activity

Source: Adapted from Leddy and Pepper (1993).

harmony can be found in holistic definitions of health and are core to
many complementary therapies.

Using the work of Fawcett, Leddy and Pepper (1993) went on to
categorise ten nursing models according to the world view they
reflected (that is, whether the model reflected the growth world view
or the stability world view). In the change-as-stability models (Table
7.1), the nature of nursing found in the five models identified is vari-
ously defined as goal orientated, an external force, a system for
promoting self-care, the manipulation of stimuli and a stress-reducing
activity. In other words, it is mainly about doing something to the
patient, force a (the nurse) acting on force b (the patient) in a one-way
transaction of cause and effect.

In contrast, the change-as-growth models (Table 7.2) describe
nursing as a therapeutic interpersonal process, transpersonal caring, the

Table 7.2   Comparison of the nature of nursing in five nursing
models classified within the change-as-growth paradigm

Nursing model	Nature of nursing
Peplau (1988)	Therapeutic interpersonal process
Watson (1985)	Transpersonal caring
Rogers (1970)	Promotion of repatterning
Newman (Marchione, 1995)	Repatterning relationships
Parse (Bunting, 1993)	Interpersonal process

Source: Adapted from Leddy and Pepper (1993).

promotion of repatterning, a repatterning partnership and an interpersonal process. In other words, nursing is about relationships not in a mechanistic way associated with cause and effect, but in a dynamic system of interaction and of realising the potential for repatterning inherent in each encounter.

The distinctions set out quite succinctly by Leddy and Pepper (1993) are helpful in clarifying some of the key debates in health care and nursing today. The first set of models (listed in Table 7.1) focus on producing and maintaining a stable steady state. The emphasis is on the skill of the practitioner in providing the right mix of treatment to control disease symptoms and maintain the patient in as healthy a condition for as long as possible. To this extent, it is possible to argue that these types of model conform to and reaffirm service-centred modes of health care delivery. They also provide an appropriate framework for workload analysis as they reproduce the central assumptions of cause and effect in nursing workload research, only in this case the situation is reversed. Rather than assuming the cause of nursing to be patient dependency and the effect nursing care, as discussed by Gault (1982) above, the cause is identified as the nursing activity and the effect the patient outcome, which could be measured as dependency (MacGuire, 1988).

The second set of models (Table 7.2) focus attention not on the interventions but on the patient. The nurses help the patients and their carers to come to terms with the disease process and learn to manage this process for themselves. In doing this, the nurse utilises whatever mix of services are necessary for patients and their carers to achieve optimal self-management of the process. The emphasis here is on recognising that the patients' understanding of the disease process will grow and develop as they learn to live with the disease. It is already known that patients frequently come to know more about specific disease trajectories than do many of the staff looking after them (Armstrong, 1984, 1987; Gull, 1987; Thorne, 1993). The change-as-growth model is about capitalising on this and facilitating the development of this process. Change as growth models can, therefore, be allied to the development of responsive patient-centred services.

The distinction between nursing as an activity that involves doing things to the patient, and nursing as an activity based on establishing a relationship with the patient, fundamentally distinguishes between two quite different ways of working in nursing. In the first case, the locus of control rests with the nurses; in the second, patients work with nurses to find a solution to their health care problem. Benner and Wrubel

(1989) describe how, in many acute settings, the first model is essential as patients and carers are often too shocked by the illness to be able to take control of the situation, and they require a skilled nurse to undertake the caring remit on their behalf. Over time, however, the situation needs to evolve and the locus of control needs to move from the nurse to the patient and his or her family.

Like centralised services, measurements and costings are much easier to derive when the locus of control rests with the nurses rather than the patients. Consequently, this aspect of nursing has been captured in nursing activity analysis and formalised in nursing workload management systems. As Leddy and Pepper highlight, this approach is also reinforced in many of the more commonly used nursing models that could form the basis of workload systems based on care planning. As Benner and Wrubel (1989) indicate, there are many situations in health care in which this approach is entirely appropriate; the problem arises when it is applied regardless of its efficacy.

Case studies and illustrative examples

The following examples are derived from a variety of recently completed research projects. All of the data were derived from interviews with patients rather than nurses, and in each case the interviews were concerned with eliciting how the patient or the primary carer felt they were managing with the illness and the type of help they felt they needed.

The data given in Vignettes 9 and 10 were all collected during a series of interviews with patients on a mixed-sex medical ward in a busy district general hospital. When asked about the nursing care on the ward, the patients whose cases are described were full of praise. The patient in Vignette 9 said, 'I couldn't fault them [(the nurses]'. The patient in Vignette 10 said:

> I specifically asked when I came in, please don't put us anywhere else but Ward X [the ward she was on] 'cos I'm so used to the nurses and I think you should go to the same ward... I mean I was in Ward Y and really I wasn't happy; I'm not saying there was anything wrong with them you know, they were lovely nurses and everything, but I missed the nurses and all them; I mean I think you feel a bit safe when you know the nurses don't you?

The data presented in these extracts illustrate that the patients were satisfied with the care they received on the ward.

Living with angina

An elderly man was admitted to hospital suffering from chest pain. He had an 18-year history of chest pain and had been forced to give up work ten years previously. He had been recommended for a triple bypass operation but had refused it, having already had one bypass operation. During the past eighteen years, this man had experienced numerous admissions to hospital with chest pain. When he was asked how the nurses on the ward managed his chest pain and whether he had been able to discuss it with them, the following conversation took place:

Patient: 'Why it's a funny thing this, at times I'm not telling them I've got a pain, 'cos I think to myself if I tell them I've got a pain, they write it down on their sheet, that might keep me in here for another day, which I'm not keen on that you na – the nurses know that and they keep on at us asking about pain and at the finish I have to tell them.'

Interviewer: 'So really you're anxious to get home as soon as possible?'

Patient: 'Oh yeah, as soon as I come in I'm anxious to get home, yeah.'

This patient had experienced numerous admissions to hospital, which he did not enjoy.

Interviewer: 'Did you call the GP out this time?'

Patient: 'Yeah, me wife did, yeah. I wasn't happy about that like, she gets herself like, I have a bit pain now, she's straight on the phone... I keep on saying to myself it'll pass... but she's not... She wants us in here to get fully checked over... cos she na's I need three bypasses done, and she na's I'm not going to have it, so terrified... I just didn't want it, I wanted to struggle on the way I is now; as long as the tablets is keeping me going, I'm happy'.

The data from the ward can be contrasted with data collected during a study funded by the English National Board for Nursing, Midwifery and Health Visiting (ENB) (ENB, 1999). The ENB study highlights a different style of working and the consequences of this different approach for the patients and their carers. In the ENB study, in-depth interviews were conducted with the informal family carers of children with chronic health problems. These were conducted in six different

Living with congestive cardiac failure

This lady had been admitted to hospital with congestive cardiac failure.

Patient: 'Well I took a, about nine months ago I had a severe heart attack you know, and the fluid filled up in me lungs a few days after and I was drowning in my own body fluid, which is horrific you know and since then this fluid keeps recurring and I can't breathe; I need the oxygen quite a lot.'

Since then the patient had experienced frequent admissions to hospital:

Patient: 'Once I get home, eh you get sick of being in here, I mean it's in and out, in and out you know; I'm never in any less than 10 days you know, getting a bit sick of it'.

Interviewer: 'How often, what sort of periods are you out for? Does it vary or…?'

Patient: 'Well it was only a fortnight this time, I think it was about five weeks the time before that, there's never been much from about October. I was like in Ward X with renal failure and then I was in Ward Y, and then I was in here and then I was back in here; you know it seems to be quite regular since the beginning of October. Its been 'cos when Dr Z [GP], he'll say oh hospital you know, I get the horrors with it you know. I've just come out and like a fortnight ago he came on the Monday and he was saying to go back to the hospital, I said I just got out yesterday; well it's a bit much isn't it?'

When asked how she managed at home, the patient said:

'When I was in the first time… 7 weeks I was in altogether… eh they did an assessment and they went to him [her husband] and saw that everything was just right a week before I went home you know, and seemingly they're going to start doing that again, but me husband's had two slight strokes and he won't have any help you know, he does it all himself and that's worrying me 'cos I think to meself, oh good God if anything happens and he collapses where are we, we're absolutely helpless.'

Interviewer: 'So they're going to do a home assessment on you before you go home this time?'

Patient: 'Well I think so… but eh I can't see where they could do really much more; I mean I've got the lift, I've got the wheelchair and all you know, so really I can't see what else they can do unless they could persuade him to have a

---

Vignette *10*

Living with congestive cardiac failure (cont'd)

home help or something like that, but he thinks that he's got to do his own as long as he's going around he's going to do it you see... He's a funny man... now he's suffering these terrible headaches, feeling sickly and headaches, and it's worrying me in case he's, you know, taking too much on himself... And then you see me keep coming back into hospital I mean from X [a town some distance away] travelling back and forwards, it's a bit much for him.'

---

geographical areas, selected for their diversity of the range and organisation of the nursing services provided to sick children.

In the ENB study, one geographical area, Area A, had established a community-based sick children's nursing service that consisted of two full-time sick children's nurses. These nurses had been instrumental in the development of the service and had provided a service that some would consider extreme and others unsustainable. The nurses were available 24 hours a day, seven days a week, including Christmas day and bank holidays. During evenings, night-times and weekends, they alternated in carrying a bleep. The parents of the sick children could contact the nurses at any time of the day or night. If the parents were concerned or having difficulty coping with a sick child who would not settle, the nurses would visit.

The mothers who had received this service spoke very highly of it, praising the nurses for the level of support. They made comments such as, 'if it hadn't been for this service, my child would have spent the first year of his life in hospital' and 'children do not only become ill between the hours of 9–5 Monday to Friday'. They talked about the importance of the relationship they developed with the nurses and how the nurses used this relationship to help the parents to gain confidence in their own clinical judgement and ability to manage the sick children. One mother said:

> They listen these nurses; they always listen to you and then they steer you in the right direction. I can be a bit hot headed, but the nurses listened and then they steered us onto a better way of managing. That's an important skill. I sometimes think people in management don't value that skill enough.

The mothers described how this was achieved: they talked about the nurses becoming 'like family members', and there was mutual respect for the contribution and knowledge that each parent and nurse had about the management of the child and the judgements of severity of a given deterioration in the child's condition.

The identification of needs within the family and the meeting of these needs by the nurses are central to many nursing theories and models. However, meeting identified needs in families might mean working in ways that do not conform to traditional nursing activities, that is, taking a child to a diabetic clinic while the mother looked after his sick brother. It requires a willingness on the part of the nurse and the service to work in ways that might not be considered to be essential nursing activities.

In another example, a health visitor looked after a baby for an afternoon while the mother caught up on her sleep. This may appear to be excessively indulgent and potentially alarming for the funders of the health service. If such a service were to be formally provided, it would probably not be considered to require the skills of a health visitor, instead being viewed as a task that could be delegated to a health care assistant. Making the offer to look after the baby informally and in response to the mother's obvious and immediate tiredness arises out of the quality of the relationship that the health visitor has been able to establish with the mother. Delegation and booking child care would overly complicate a simple human response. Moreover, the mother might not be happy to leave her baby with someone she has not got to know.

The importance of relationships in underpinning responsive provision, as highlighted in nursing models that focus on change as growth, seems central to this way of working. In such scenarios, it seems that the strength of the growth achieved through the relationship may derive from the sharing of the menial tasks, the exchange of skills in the management of menial tasks and the development of trust and mutual respect that evolves from sharing these tasks together.

Interestingly, the accounts given by the mothers who experienced the nursing service offered in Area A affirmed these suggestions. Their accounts seemed to indicate that, far from increasing the demand, the intervention of the nurses at a very early stage in the crisis appeared to prevent further deterioration and keep the children at home and out of hospital. When called out, the nurses shared in the care 'as if they were a family member', undertaking any family tasks that were necessary, including looking after other children. It was this approach that was appreciated by the parents. It appeared to enable them to cope and gave them confidence, making the stress of caring for the child manageable and possibly preventing an escalation in stress to the point at which the intervention of social services in the form of foster care became necessary.

The nurses providing the service in Area A were clearly highly skilled. An unsuccessful management of this approach to nursing could lead to the creation of excessive dependency on the nurses, who could then undertake an increasing burden of family care. Moreover, if the nurses did not fully appreciate the way in which they were working, they could find it difficult to refuse demands and become overwhelmed by the complexity of the issues with which they were dealing, finding it difficult if not impossible to identify any boundaries on provision. Moreover, the service could be very costly depending on the level of demand, and it might be difficult to identify these costs in advance of demand. This type of service provision could also have a detrimental effect on the family and social lives of the nurses themselves, making recruitment into this type of service difficult to achieve.

The examples from the ENB study illustrate that there are different ways of working in nursing, and these ways of working can have a profound effect on the coping strategies of families dealing with illness. In Vignettes 9 and 10, it is clear that while the nurses on the medical ward were providing care that was held in high esteem by patients, the conceptual models of nursing that they were using conformed to the change-as-stability model of nursing. In other words, in keeping with most nursing emanating from hospital-based provision, the emphasis was on the stabilisation of the patient's condition within the confines of the hospital and in isolation from the context of the social situation to which they were to be discharged.

Vignette 9 is particularly interesting from this point of view. If a nurse could establish a good enough relationship with the patient's wife, such that she were prepared to call the nurse rather than an ambulance the next time the patient experienced severe chest pain, and the nurse was able to stay with the family until the pain had subsided, teaching the wife, over a number of episodes, how to monitor the severity of the episode, then the number of repeat admissions to hospital experienced by this patient might be radically reduced. As the interview extract indicates, this would greatly increase his quality of life and also reduce the anxiety experienced by his wife every time he had a chest pain.

These descriptors of nursing practice reflect findings from other studies. Bottorff (1997) describes work undertaken in Canada into promoting autonomy within dependency for patients requiring palliative care. She describes the types of choices that patients make in relation to personal and nursing care routines, including when to get out of bed, how long to stay up and whether to take a bath or a shower. For those who are physically fit, these decisions may appear trivial as bodily functions may be a minor consideration. For palliative care patients, however, new ways to live in the world have to be found that reduce or prevent the domination of the person's life by his or her body. In such circumstances, the ways in which patients and their families learn to manage bodily functions is fundamental to their quality of life.

Nursing is clearly fundamental to this process. The brief debate of nursing theories and models, and the distinctions drawn by Fawcett (1989) and Leddy and Pepper (1993), illustrate different approaches to nursing. The identification of different approaches raises the need for further research into the cost–benefits of using different models of service provision.

The data collected in the ENB study do not permit the identification of a causal relationship between the successful outcome found in the data for those families cared for by the nurses in Area A compared to outcomes in other parts of the country where this type of service has not been developed. A more systematic approach to research over a prolonged period of time is required to elicit fully the real effects on the health of families and their children of different models of nursing service provision. This type of research would provide a much sounder basis for identifying the number of nurses needed and the skill mix required linked to patient and family outcomes than does the contemporary emphasis on the minute-by-minute activity analysis prevalent in so many nursing workload studies.

The above examples highlight the need to develop a less descriptive and more systematic approach to nursing research in workforce planning that undertakes a comparative analysis of different theoretical nursing models and tests out the effectiveness of these models with different client groups. This requires the development of operational and user-friendly definitions of the nursing theories listed by Leddy and Pepper (1993). It also requires developing nurse practitioners who understand these definitions and who are adequately resourced and committed to working with and developing these theories at least for the duration of the research. Evidence of the short-, medium- and long-term impact of different ways of working with patients in terms of their ability to cope successfully with the consequences of the illness could then be collected.

Measuring and timing tasks performed by nurses will never supply the organisation with information pertinent to the successful or unsuccessful resolution of the issues illustrated above. Should services fail to address issues such as the care of relatives while primary carers are hospitalised, or the resolution of the anxieties of primary carers, they will not register, except perhaps as a complaint or as a covert failure to comply with the best available treatment or report relevant symptoms.

Vignettes 9 and 10 illustrate the potential health gains of customising services to take account of or be responsive to the individual circumstances of patients. This may involve taking a more proactive role in helping family and informal carers to learn about the way in which they are caring for the patient, and the impact that this has on the patient's experience of the illness, as well as the health and well-being of the carer. Undertaking a more proactive stance in helping the carer to care could be viewed as intrusive and invasive of family privacy. It could also reflect the fact that caring is a skilled and complex activity that has to be learnt and may not evolve naturally just from the experience of being a carer.

MacGuire's (1988) work illustrates how the creation of dependency is an inherent aspect of caring relationships. Consequently, allowing care to evolve naturally within the patient–lay carer relationship is likely to result in the creation of dependency rather than independence, thus increasing the care burden and the collective costs to society of meeting this burden of care (Royal Commission on Long Term Care, 1999). Nolan and Grant (1989) highlight how informal and lay carers frequently and persistently request just this type of support and experience considerable difficulty in accessing it. Benner and Wrubel (1989) point out that if the complex knowledge base of caring is acknowledged, caring ceases to be a burden and becomes a challenging and fulfilling aspect of human existence.

Summary and conclusion

This chapter has reviewed the extensive literature on nurse workforce planning. It has highlighted conceptual and methodological problems with mainstream studies in this area. In particular, it has demonstrated how the findings from such studies reflect professional ideologies about care needs rather than evidence-based outcomes.

The distinctive approaches to nursing described by Leddy and Pepper (1993) are highlighted because they provide an opportunity to conceptualise different approaches to nursing care. This creates a situation in which it is possible to compare the adoption of each approach for its effect on the health outcome for patients and their families and the cost of providing different types of nursing service. Using theory as depicted by Leddy and Pepper (1993) could give rise to the development of nursing workload tools that adopt a theoretical definition of nursing, as against the current descriptive definition. The strength of this is that the data collected would be directly linked to the theoretical perspective identified in the tool. It is this which would be measured and used to establish the nurse staffing levels.

It is probable that, in their practice, nurses use the full range of approaches encompassed in nursing models. By developing theoretically based nursing workload management tools, Trusts could choose which aspects of nursing they wished to capture as a basis for determining the staffing establishment. The decision of which tool to adopt could be based on principles and philosophies of Trust provision as set out in mission statements, or it could be based on evidence derived from research indicating the approach to nursing that is most cost-effective in relation to identified patient outcomes. These could in turn be informed by the definitions of health described in Chapter 2. The use of theoretically based tools would also enable a valid comparison to be made between organisations, so that the current situation of trying to compare dissimilar services, highlighted by the Audit Commission (1991), would be avoided.

So finally, evidence is required in nursing, but this evidence does not necessarily need more rigour as most of the research into nursing workload systems has been highly rigorous in its own terms. Instead, nursing evidence actually needs more theory, an analysis based not on tasks but on the effectiveness of tasks in achieving agreed patient outcomes, and on the decision making processes required to link the task to the desired patient outcome.

To provide a final example, the task of providing a bedpan, a most fundamental task in nursing, will be discussed. In providing access to toilet facilities, patient choice is central, but nursing resources and the skill mix available may circumscribe the range of choice. Rehabilitating the patient by assisting him or her to walk may require more than one nurse, yet a bedpan or commode may be provided by just one nurse. How the dilemma of enabling the patient to access toilet facilities is resolved in the face of inadequate staffing turns on whether the nurse recognises the opportunity of giving the patient a choice between options arising from the resources available, and in so doing promoting and facilitating patient problem solving.

Arguably, the ability to solve problems such as these will be essential outside the confines of the hospital. It also requires both the nurse and the patient to be aware of the safe parameters within which this choice could be realised. For some patients, this may not be an issue, but for others it may be a crucial part of learning to live with the illness. Making this type of distinction enables systematic research to be undertaken based on theoretically different approaches to nursing provision and the impact of these approaches on patients. If these distinctions can be realised in practice, there is a real possibility of undertaking a cost–benefit analysis of skill mix in nursing related to health outcomes derived from theoretically different nursing approaches.

Chapter 8

Managing Demand through Care

Chapter 3 highlighted the enduring concerns about the escalating cost of health care bought about by a variety of factors including the ageing of the population, the increasing sophistication of medical technology and the rise in consumer demand and expectations. Figure 3.2 outlined two models of health care provision: a selective model of provision and a universal model of provision. This chapter extends the discussion of these two models and links the two models to different approaches to demand management in health care.

As described in Chapter 3, the selective model focuses on cost containment by introducing barriers to access and reducing the length of patient contact with services. The universal approach recognises that, in a policy arena where free access to services on demand via general practice or A&E services forms the founding principle for the provision of many Western health services, for example the NHS (DoH, 1996b), patient behaviour will ultimately determine demand. Patient behaviour is, however, not independent of service provision. Instead, the ways in which patients learn to manage illness and to use services arises, in part, from the way in which those services are provided. There is an interactive element between patient behaviour and service provision, the processes of which will be fundamental in determining the level of demand that patients make on services.

This chapter thus provides a discussion of selective and universal approaches to demand management and locates each approach within a broader debate on sources of professional knowledge, information management, skill mix and professional accountability, focusing specifically on emerging debates on these issues in the nursing literature.

The influence of the medical model on health service provision

It is generally recognised that the introduction of the NHS in 1948 was based on a number of assumptions about the nature of health care. One assumption was that universal provision of health services would lead to a reduction in demand as it would conquer at least one of Beveridge's 'Five Giants' – that of disease (Barnard, 1977).

The notion of conquering disease or curing illness has dominated health care provision ever since. It is, as numerous writers point out, fundamental to the medical model of health. For example, Osherson and AmaraSingham (1981) suggest that medicine has increasingly conceptualised the body as a machine made up of component parts that can be examined and treated in isolation from one another and from the rest of the body. Similarly, Seedhouse (1986) points out that medicine is based on the assumption that the best way to cure disease is to reduce bodies to their constituent parts and treat the diseased part rather than the ill person.

Both Seedhouse (1986) and Osherson and AmaraSingham (1981) suggest that the domination of medical science by the machine metaphor gives rise to the view that health is a commodity that can be supplied by the application of appropriate technical interventions following the onset of disease. Within this conceptualisation of health and illness, health is defined as the absence of disease. Health, for an ill person, can only be achieved by curing the underlying disease process. It is possible to argue that this definition of health has dominated health care policy since the inception of the NHS and goes some way towards accounting for the invisibility of holistic approaches to health in health policy literature.

Putting users' and carers' needs first

The phrase 'putting users' and carers' needs first' is derived from the Audit Commission report on community services (Audit Commission, 1992). This report recognises that the traditional organisational framework for health service provision has become a major impediment to the development of services that meet the needs of the users. The Audit Commission recognises that, for this to be addressed, health services provision must adopt a new method of working. The traditional and new methods of working identified by the Audit Commission are depicted in Figure 8.1.

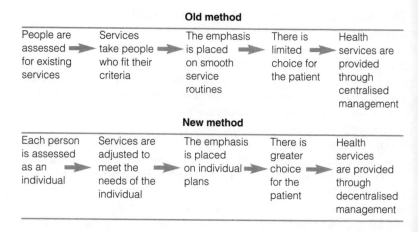

Figure 8.1 'Putting users' and carers' needs first' – old and new methods of working in health care provision
Source: Adapted from Audit Commission (1992).

The second approach has been endorsed in the UK publication *Partnership in Action: New Opportunities for Joint Working between Health and Social Services* (DoH, 1998a), which states that government proposals for the NHS 'will put the needs of users and carers firmly at the centre of health and social service provision' (p. 8). This shift in policy challenges many of the current practices that constitute political and status relationships within the NHS.

A central preoccupation of contemporary health care systems is the need to contain costs in the face of spiralling medical technology (McLachlan, 1990). Consequently, attempts to implement changes in organisational structure and service provision require evidence of both the efficacy and the effectiveness of the proposed service. The development of information technology and the opportunity to analyse large data sets has given rise to the concept of evidence-based health care planning (DoH, 1998d). Contrary to the Audit Commission, which argues for decentralised management, Maynard (1994) recommends greater managerial control over the decision-making processes of health care professionals in order to promote the most effective use of resources.

There is, therefore, a dilemma at the heart of government policy. On the one hand, the need to decentralise services in order to respond effectively to the individual needs of users has been recognised by the Audit Commission, but control over the decisions of professionals is seen as paramount if the costs of the service are to be contained.

The impact of sources of knowledge on the structure of health care provision

Chapter 3 demonstrated that medical science has made some progress in combating disease, but much of this progress centres on symptom management rather than cure of diseases that are characterised by a degenerative trajectory. In degenerative disease management, clinical effectiveness requires patients as well as professionals to undertake evidenced-based practice in their daily management of the disease process. Promoting clinically effective patients remains an unresolved issue within the current organisation of care provision (Kaplun, 1992; Thorne, 1993).

It follows, therefore, that in order to develop clinical effectiveness, professional knowledge has to be successfully integrated with patient/family and community knowledge. This requires that medical knowledge derived from the physical sciences be integrated with the use of knowledge and the development of services derived from the social sciences.

In this context, Leininger's (1988) theory of transcultural nursing provides an interesting example of how this might be achieved. Leininger (1988) introduced the concept of 'transcultural nursing' to highlight the complex problems associated with implementing health care for culturally diverse populations. The theory of transcultural nursing originated in the USA, where health care professionals are highly likely to encounter people with an ethnic and racial background different from their own. Leininger argued that an awareness of the impact of culture on the patient is necessary if nurses are to provide culturally appropriate care.

According to Boyle and Andrews (1989), the theory of transcultural nursing is derived from a synthesis of concepts borrowed from anthropology, sociology and biology, combined with the nursing concepts of caring, nursing process and interpersonal communications. The focus of transcultural nursing is on deriving an agreement between the nurse and the patient on the meaning of certain cultural symbols, such as health, healing, illness, disease and caring.

This enables the nurse to respond to the patient in ways that fully support the patient's cultural integrity, allowing the patient to maintain his or her own values, norms, beliefs and traditions. Different cultural behaviours exhibited by patients should be viewed as assets rather than liabilities. Reaching agreement with the patient over the meaning of cultural phenomena in relation to health enables the nurse to reframe problems in order to support health behaviours without expecting patients to give up their unique cultural inheritance. This description of nursing very much mirrors the discussion of nursing given in Chapter 4, where it was suggested that good nursing practice is about identifying and responding to patients' needs in a non-coercive environment.

The concept of transcultural nursing, in focusing on maintaining the cultural integrity of the patient, overlaps with Kitson's (1993) depiction of nursing in which care is defined as ethical position, and Benner and Wrubel's (1989) depiction of care as differentiating and identifying what is important within the context of the situation. This is discussed in more detail in Chapter 5.

In contrast, the overriding concern to cure disease that characterises medicine (Osherson and AmaraSingham, 1981; Thorne, 1993) creates a tendency for physicians to distrust patients' views of their own experience in favour of statistically derived evidence. Patients' problems with struggling to integrate the demands of medical regimes with the integrity of their cultural heritage remain unrecognised. Instead, health professionals regard the multiple pressures of daily living experienced by patients and their families as obstacles to compliance. Health care professionals are unable to recognise and respond to the real dilemmas confronting patients in complying with clinically effective medical regimes (Coates and Boore, 1996; Watson, 1998), giving rise to Thorne and Robinson's concept of guarded alliance (Thorne and Robinson, 1989), described in Chapter 4. As Leddy and Pepper (1993) point out, cultural phenomena (values and behaviour), within the tradition of the health service, that do not reflect the predominant values and expected behaviours of the health service could be viewed as a liability.

This would appear to be the case under the traditional approach to health care provision described by the Audit Commission (1992) and illustrated in Figure 8.1 above. As depicted by the Audit Commission, people are assessed for existing services, and services admit only those people who fit the service criteria. Non-compliance with a treatment offered would, under this system, be grounds for rejecting the patient as being inappropriate for the service provided. The provision of services based upon narrow cultural criteria is likely to be inappropriate for sections of the population with different cultural backgrounds. Consequently, those individuals or populations who do not meet the criteria for care enshrined in existing service provision will not be catered for and will be disenfranchised.

The switch from traditional approaches to service provision depicted by the Audit Commission, to the decentralised approach advocated, could be aligned to the movement from a provision of services based on the natural (physical) sciences to a service based on knowledge derived from the social sciences. The problem confronting the health service in bringing about this change is to assume that knowledge derived from the social sciences can be applied in exactly the same way as knowledge derived from the physical sciences. The brief discussion of transcultural nursing given above illustrates the complexity of using social science-based knowledge. It is doubtful whether such knowledge could be processed and disseminated via the medium of expert systems or clinical guidelines, as in the example of the use of aspirin to reduce the risk of a heart attack (NHS Centre for Reviews and Dissemination, 1995).

Health services are faced with the challenge of integrating knowledge derived from the physical sciences with knowledge derived from the social sciences when taking forward evidenced-based care. This integration is required in order to enable patients and their families to become clinically effective at managing disease processes while simultaneously maintaining their cultural and individual integrity.

Managing costs and escalating demands for health care

The development of evidence-based knowledge derived from the physical sciences is increasingly being linked via the process of therapeutic interventions to 'expert management systems' of the type envisioned by Spurgeon (1993). Spurgeon describes the implementation of a modern integrated hospital information system. The system depicts an efficient method of meeting the patient's immediate physiological needs. Through the integrated system, beds are managed, drugs are ordered and stocks replenished, pathology tests are requested, specimens are dispatched in labelled bottles, and the results are transmitted to the appropriate ward. Bed availability is monitored, and beds are located to meet fluctuating demands.

From the description given, research-based therapeutic interventions derived from knowledge grounded in the physical sciences become the substance of the 'expert system'. The professionals can, via the integrated management system, be given up-to-date knowledge to enhance their clinical decision making, while at the same time their activities can be monitored to ensure compliance with the expert system. This type of approach has been advocated as an effective method of implementing evidence-based practice in medicine (Grimshaw and Russell, 1993).

The costs of the service are calculated using a combination of epidemiological data on illness profiles linked to appropriate therapeutic interventions identified in the expert system and to the capacity of the service to respond to local needs. Thus, the system ensures not only that patients receive the most up-to-date care, but also that the costs of this care can be calculated and maintained within predetermined cash limits. This is a central preoccupation of contemporary health care systems (McLachlan, 1990).

Within the scenario of expert evidence-based systems dominated by approaches to knowledge derived from the physical sciences, the work of nurses becomes increasingly more complex and marginalised. The technological efficiency depicted in the integrated management system described by Spurgeon (1993) creates considerable work for nurses. Nurses have to ensure that patients understand what is happening to them and why, as well as to address any anxieties and fears that patients may have about their illness and the response of the hospital to it this time as against on a previous admission. This has to be undertaken in a series of short bursts as the patient moves from A&E through a series of specialist departments (for example, the medical admissions ward, the general medical ward and the discharge ward), according to the availability of beds and the priorities allocated to bed utilisation. Consequently, patients may only stay a few hours or days in each department.

This approach secures efficient throughput in terms of hospital statistics, and increased productivity, for each department involved and for the hospital as a whole, justifying the continued existence of the system. It does not, however, enable health service staff in general and nurses in particular to develop a shared understanding with patients of the nature of their illness and the meaning it holds for them. Instead, nurses are busy completing the numerous computerised forms generated by the system and devising ever more complex communication strategies with all the professional staff involved in the care of the patient, necessary to ensure the smooth transfer of the patient from one department to the next.

The transfer of care has to be completed with all the legal documentation intact and with all the professional staff involved in care aware of the location of the patient at the particular time when they wish to undertake a therapeutic intervention or provide a service. The intervention could be physiotherapy, an investigation such as a blood test or X-ray, or a drug prescription, while the service could be domestic, for example ensuring that patients have the meal they ordered rather than one destined for the bed's previous occupant. The more depersonalised the system becomes, as managers strive for greater technological efficiency and output, the harder the nurses have to work to explain the complexity of the system to the patient. At the same time, the co-ordinating role of nursing is emphasised as nurses are required to manage the complexity to ensure the smooth progression of the patient through the increasing range of specialist services.

The impact of organisational change designed to improve hospital efficiency has been reviewed by McKee *et al.* (1998). They cite evidence from the USA and Canada suggesting that a low level of hospital nurse satisfaction is most closely associated with a perceived heavy workload and difficulty in communication. Further evidence indicates that nurse satisfaction is a good predictor of quality of care, a low level of nurse satisfaction correlating closely with a higher level of in-patient mortality. McKee *et al.* conclude that, in the absence of information on the impact of organisational change on the quality of care and on patient outcome, coupled with the use of measurable indicators such as cost rather than patient-centred criteria, there is a danger that hospitals could become pressure chambers rather than safe spaces for clinical care.

This could be reinforced if integrated management systems continue to respond to the patient as an event rather than a person. Although the system might identify that the patient has been admitted before, a concern to maximise bed utilisation tends to override the use of details of past relationships with hospital staff as a factor in deciding the management of the patient's care.

The development of integrated expert management systems may secure the efficient processing of patients through hospital facilities and the allocation of increasingly accurate costings to aid hospital budgeting, but the relationship between this approach to care management and definitions of health is much more problematic. The continued domination of health care by knowledge derived and validated by using methods associated with the physical sciences continues the tradition of professional dominance (Freidson, 1970). The patient remains a passive recipient of, albeit expert, care. Expert management systems, therefore, retain the elevated status of technological interventions over other models of care management.

Such a position can be justified in situations where the research evidence points unequivocally to cure as a realisable outcome of the technological intervention. The emphasis on evidence-based 'expert systems' is, however, less obvious in cases where cure is not yet a realisable goal, or where the knowledge underpinning the expert system is derived primarily from the social as against the natural or physical sciences. This is the case in health promotion, public health, preventative health care and the management of chronic degenerative diseases.

The technological solution depicted above fails to achieve continuity or responsibility for the overall care management of the patient. No single person or team of people is responsible for the management of the patient. The hospital retains an elevated status over community medicine, but there is no incentive or long-term responsibility for facilitating optimum patient control over the course of the illness under current arrangements for managing care in the hospital sector. This was found to be one of the most enduring problems preventing the effective discharge from hospital of patients who were predicted to be at risk of unsuccessful discharge (Pearson *et al.*, 1998).

Instead, the system creates a process of continual referral in response to physiological indicators and service availability that renders the patient a passive recipient of care and the staff as processors of treatment protocols. Concepts of transcultural nursing described above indicate the need to develop a shared understanding between the staff and the patient in order to facilitate patient control over the illness and maintain patient integrity. Such a process remains, along with the nursing staff, marginalised from the hospital system.

From an organisational perspective, constant referral prevents any one group of staff taking overall responsibility for the progress and adaptive response of the patient. From a personal perspective, the humanitarian concern of health service staff for individual patients and their plight becomes more difficult to sustain with a decreasing length of stay and a high level of referral and throughput. This gives rise to segmented inputs in which the only people who have a complete overview of the patients' experience are the patients themselves, whose knowledge is deemed to be marginal within an evidence-based ideology.

From an experiential perspective, the opportunity to learn how to help patients in a holistic manner to confront the complexity of their illness is lost. The input of individual staff is dissipated and contact is either brief or subservient to the decisions of more senior staff, who, while technically excellent, have little opportunity for sustained patient contact or for learning about the consequences of their input and its long-term effect on the patient's overall well-being.

In addressing the issue of providing patient-centred services, health service managers have to confront the problem of distinguishing the use of 'evidence' to control professionals from the use of 'evidence' to control patients. If services are provided on the basis of evidence derived predominantly from the physical sciences alone, the health service will continue treating only patients who fit existing service criteria. The need to tailor services to the individual needs of patients, as recommended by the Audit Commission, will fail to materialise.

In the light of this discussion, it is possible to suggest two alternatives for managing the escalating demand for health care in the face of an ageing population and a disease profile dominated by chronic illness. The first approach manages demand by reducing access to hospital services; the second approach reduces demand by working with patients and their family or informal carers to resolve problems.

Model 1: Managing demand by selective policies designed to reduce access to hospital services

In the selective approach, demand is managed by transferring hospital services into the community, decreasing access to hospitals, increasing hospital throughput and reducing the length of hospital stay. There is considerable evidence that this is the approach that has been adopted over most of Europe and North America (US Congress Office of Technology Assessment, 1995; WHO, 1997b).

Within health care, medical technology is managed in hospitals, which continue to consume the largest proportion of health care spending (US Congress Office of Technology Assessment, 1995). In undertaking their review of organisational change and the quality of health care from an international perspective, McKee *et al.*, (1998) identified three change strategies designed to reduce access to hospitals. The first seeks to shift patients currently treated in hospital into other care settings. The second seeks to reconfigure the way in which hospitals provide care by, for example, altering skill mix and reducing length of stay. The third seeks to review the overall provision of hospital services to a given population. In each of these scenarios, the aim is to reduce or contain the overall cost of health care. As McKee *et al.* (1998) point out, there is very little evidence to suggest that these strategies will reduce health care costs, and their impact on quality of care and patient outcome is largely unknown.

It is arguably the case that this approach reinforces the supremacy of knowledge derived from the physical sciences over knowledge derived from the social sciences in health care provision. Increasing cost is met by substituting medical staff for nursing staff, reducing the number of qualified nurses, increasing the number of unqualified nurses and making increasing use of bank and agency staff. This scenario has been identified in a review of trends in the nursing workforce in the UK, commissioned by the UKCC (Warner *et al.*, 1998).

This report identified something of a polarisation in nursing skills. At one end of the spectrum, there was evidence of a trend towards substituting qualified nurses with lesser trained staff. At the other, a trend towards the recruitment and development of a small number of highly qualified nursing staff with considerable professional autonomy and the expertise to undertake medical tasks such as prescribing medication could be discerned.

Such an approach is unlikely to reduce demand, but it may contain cost as demand rises. Evidence provided by Prescott (1993), McKenna (1995) and McKee *et al.* (1998) suggests that attempts to reduce hospital costs rarely focus on a reduction in the purchase or use of medical technology, despite evidence that medical technology is largely responsible for escalating costs and has only a marginal impact on health gain, one that falls far short of the level of resources currently invested in it (Abel-Smith, 1994). Instead, the size of the workforce makes nursing the biggest single item in any health care provider's budget and therefore a target for cost improvement programmes. This is despite considerable evidence, cited by Prescott, McKenna and McKee *et al.*, that high-quality nursing care reduces the demand for medical technology by increasing the self-care agency of the patient, and in turn lowers overall the health care cost.

Model 2: Managing demand by universal policies designed to work with patients and family/informal carers to resolve problems

The universal approach to managing demand for health care recognises that patients are proactive in their help-seeking behaviour. Hospital admission is triggered by a crisis that provides an opportunity to engage with the family and the patient to review self-care strategies, social support networks and the family management of care to promote health (Connelly, 1987; Gull, 1987; Newby, 1996).

Evidence for this second approach can be found in studies into the effective discharge of patients from hospital in which a specific, trained, clinical member of staff takes responsibility for the discharge process (Neidlinger *et al.*, 1987; Naylor, 1990; Moher *et al.*, 1992; Houghton *et al.*, 1996; Runciman *et al.*, 1996; Morris *et al.*, 1997). All of these studies describe the benefits of a well-planned and co-ordinated discharge process. In each case, a named professional, usually educated to at least graduate and frequently post-graduate level, takes responsibility for co-ordinating care and communicating with all parties involved in the process across the primary–secondary care interface, including the patients and their carers. In these studies, both the number of admissions to hospital and the number of days spent in hospital were reduced, creating a true reduction in demand for hospital care rather than merely containing escalating demand by reducing the average cost per patient day.

Here, it is suggested that service provision adopts a holistic problem-solving approach in which intensive care and support are provided in the most appropriate setting to resolve the underlying difficulties. The effect of such an approach is again largely unknown as few services are developed according to these criteria. There is some evidence, from Canada, that proactive, preventative community care reduces the cost to the whole system while sustaining patients at a similar level of phys-ical functioning (Browne *et al.*, 1994).

It would appear, however, that, in keeping with current approaches to health care management, most nurse staffing and nurse budget setting is informed by the selective approaches to demand management described above. Here, the efficacy of an increasingly unqualified nursing workforce is reinforced within a demand-led service in which the emphasis is on containing rather than resolving patient care prob-lems. As the number of people experiencing health care problems grows, it is likely that the cost of containment will similarly increase, precipitating a search for ever cheaper forms of containment.

Skill mix in nursing and health care

Skill mix and labour substitution are enduring and evolving issues in health care. For nursing, these present a continual challenge in which pressure is applied for nurses to undertake an increasing range of tasks previously carried out by medical staff while simultaneously delegating an increasing range of nursing care to unqualified support workers (Dickinson, 1982; Warner, *et al.*, 1998).

As the previous chapter demonstrated, the issue of the number of qualified nurses required to provide nursing services and the skill mix of those services, remains, despite considerable research, a contentious and unresolved issue. McKenna (1995), in a review of nursing skill mix substitution and quality of nursing care, identified three central assumptions that govern decision making on skill mix substitution in nursing. The first of these suggests that a rich skill mix of mostly qualified nurses is often an ineffective and inefficient way of providing health care. The second assumption is based on evidence suggesting that a skill mix of mostly unqualified staff is an ineffective approach to health care provision. The third proposes that the most effective and efficient way in which to provide health care is to employ a high number of qualified nurses.

These three assumptions map onto the development of nursing care described by Kitson and discussed in Chapter 5. According to Kitson (1993), care in nursing has evolved from care-as-duty through care-as-therapeutic-action to care-as-ethical-position. McKenna's first assumption, that employing qualified nurses is an ineffective and inefficient way of providing health care, is likely to give rise to nursing within the care-as-duty paradigm, as depicted in the first approach to demand management described above. Here, nursing will be characterised by undifferentiated routines and procedures as a predominantly unqualified nursing workforce will exercise only limited clinical autonomy.

The second of McKenna's assumptions suggests that a balance between unqualified and qualified nurses needs to be established. This assumption seems to reflect the current position in nursing in the UK identified by the UKCC (Warner *et al.*, 1998). Here, an increasing polarisation of the nursing workforce was identified, a cadre of highly qualified nurses taking on an increasing amount of professional autonomy and responsibility for therapeutic interventions. The UKCC analysis maps on to Kitson's notion of care-as-therapeutic-position, although it is recognised that it extends Kitson's definition of therapeutics to include delegated medical interventions such as prescribing, suturing and other medical procedures. Where this departs from Kitson's analysis is in delegating an increasing range of nursing care to an unqualified workforce.

Finally, McKenna's third assumption, about the efficacy of a rich skill mix in nursing comprising predominantly qualified nurses, reflects Kitson's description of care-as-ethical-position. Care-as-ethical-position recognises the decision-making components embedded in everyday nursing care activities and seeks to ensure that those delivering nursing care have the expertise to take decisions that will resolve rather than contain or exacerbate patient care problems.

Role substitution and ambiguity in nursing work

The role boundaries between the work of qualified and unqualified nurses have long been a contentious issue in nursing (DHSS, 1982a; Dickinson, 1982; Coveney, 1983;). Much of the debate has revolved around attempts to distinguish those tasks which can be performed by unqualified nurses from tasks which remain the prerogative of qualified nurses. This difficulty arises from the assumption that a high proportion of the tasks undertaken by nurses are relatively simple and do not require a substantial amount of training or education to perform them effectively. This interpretation of nursing work was certainly predominant up until the end of the 1980s. Menzies (1960), for example, suggests that 'the nursing service must face the dilemma that, while a strong sense of responsibility and discipline are felt to be necessary for the welfare of patients, a considerable proportion of actual nursing tasks are extremely simple (p. 21). Similarly, Fretwell (1982), in a study of learning opportunities for students when they formed part of the nursing workforce, suggested that greater learning opportunities existed when students were involved in technical care, proposing this has a decision-making component not found in 'basic' care routines.

Nursing has traditionally been divided into three broad categories of work. 'Basic' care refers to the more personalised areas of nursing such as bathing, feeding, mobilising and toileting patients. The second category, technical care, refers to curative interventions and includes wound dressing and the care of intravenous infusions. The third category is administrative care or management that involves ward organisation, the co-ordination of care and ensuring an adequate supply of equipment and drugs. This classification of nursing work was used by Goddard (1953) as a basis for developing workload indicators in nursing and remained the predominant framework for analysing nursing work for many years.

The focus on tasks arising out of this classification of nursing work perpetuated an understanding of nursing work as predominantly unskilled work. However, numerous studies found in practice that although unqualified staff might predominantly give 'basic' nursing care, it was rarely given exclusively by these staff. For example, Hardie (1978), in an investigation of auxiliary nurse training courses, found 'that all the task areas covered in the registered nurse syllabus of the General Nursing Council, with the exception of injections and certain forms of drainage, are carried out somewhere in the UK by auxiliaries' (p. 47).

More recently, Workman (1996), in a qualitative investigation into how health care assistants perceive their role as 'support workers' to qualified staff, found considerable role ambiguity between health care assistants and qualified nurses. Again, some health care assistants stated that they did everything a qualified nurse did in relation to the provision of patient care. Workman suggests that qualified nurses appear to lack clarity with regard to their own role and that this affects their expectations of health care assistants. She recommends greater clarity over role expectations in order to reduce role ambiguity and alleviate the stress that this appears to cause qualified nurses and health care assistants alike.

What is apparent from the above debate on the distribution of nursing work between qualified and unqualified nursing staff is the focus on tasks rather than decision making. To this end, the debate does not appear to have moved from Kitson's first paradigm of nursing that emphasises care-as-duty. The knowledge-based decision-making aspects of nursing identified in Kitson's other two paradigms have not been utilised to inform the skill mix debate in nursing.

Accountability in nursing care

The distinction between tasks and decision making has a long history in nursing. The debate was traditionally based on the assumption that decision making about care could be retained by the qualified nurse while the tasks emanating from the decisions could be delegated to less well qualified nurses who would provide the care within agreed parameters and procedures. This is the definition of autonomy given by Batey and Lewis (1982, p. 15), who define autonomy as 'the freedom to make discretionary and binding decisions consistent with one's scope of practice and freedom to act on those decisions'. In their discussion of accountability, they suggest that professional accountability derives from the authority of expert knowledge. The authority of expert knowledge suggest that individuals exercise authority as a result of the personal attributes (skills and expertise) that they possess and that are a prerequisite for being given a post.

Accountability based on expert knowledge is, therefore, dependent on the skill of the person rather than on the authority vested by an organisation in a given post such as 'head of department'. It thus follows that the authority of the post cannot be delegated as it is derived from the expertise of the individual. According to Batey and Lewis (1982), while the authority of the expert cannot be delegated, it is possible to delegate the charges or responsibilities emanating from the post. In such circumstances, it is they rather than the person to whom the actions are delegated who retains accountability for the consequences of delegated actions.

Batey and Lewis's discussion of professional accountability turns, therefore, on the authority to take decisions. If there is no authority to take decisions on the content of nursing work, then, according to Batey and Lewis, there can be no accountability. A person can be held accountable only if he or she takes a decision about work content, and then only for the consequences of the aspect of work related to this decision.

The description of professional accountability given by Batey and Lewis (1982) accords with what Melia (1995) has described as bureaucratic organisational structures. Melia suggests that any group that provides a complex service for society will do so through a bureaucratic organisational structure in which the roles and lines of accountability are clearly defined. As Melia points out, line management works precisely through lines of accountability. The bureaucratic organisational chart indicates who is accountable to whom for what. However, as Melia suggests, while the notion of accountability provides the diagram for the delivery of services, the content or quality of the service delivered depends upon the responsibility that the individual takes for the action.

According to Melia, being responsible carries with it the freedom of moral agency during the space of time when an individual is carrying out the activities for which he or she is accountable. Using this interpretation of accountability, the distinction between accountability and delegation made by Batey and Lewis (1982) cannot be sustained. All individuals are accountable for the way in which they undertake their delegated duties and do this through the exercise of responsibility.

In nursing, much of the activity is invisible and known only to the patient and the nurse (Lawler, 1991; Melia, 1995). Consequently, it may be possible to say that so many patients have been bathed, fed or given medication, but this provides very little information on the nature of the activity or the way in which it was conducted. Melia emphasises that the way in which nurses of all grades exercise responsibility in relation to individual care activities constitutes both the quality and the outcome of nursing care.

From Melia's analysis of accountability and responsibility in nursing care, it follows that the concept of accountability applies to all nurses, be they qualified or unqualified. This does not necessarily, however, imply the employment of an all-qualified workforce. It simply highlights the limitations of adopting an overly bureaucratic approach to nurse management in which the quality of care is located in procedures, protocols and the delegation of tasks rather than in the recognition of and support for the exercise of responsibility by all members of the nursing workforce.

Accountability in primary nursing

The issue of accountability in nursing has been thrown into sharp relief by the introduction of primary nursing (Manthey, 1980). Primary nursing is a system of nursing in which each individual patient is allocated a primary named nurse. That nurse is accountable for the patient's care for the duration of time the patient is on the ward or unit. The nurse is responsible for developing the care plan for the 24-hour period, including identifying care needs during any off-duty time. An associate nurse is responsible for providing care in accordance with the care plan when the primary nurse is off duty. Primary nursing depends on a flattened hierarchical structure so that nurses can have autonomy and authority over the care of individual patients (Rodgers, 1995).

In primary nursing, overall accountability for care lies with the primary nurse, but all nurses providing care are responsible for adhering to the care plan and providing care in such a way as to promote the planned outcome of care. A care plan aimed at rehabilitating a patient who has suffered a stroke, for example, may require nurses to teach and motivate the patient to undertake self-care activities such as washing and feeding. The patient may complain about the difficulty of doing these tasks and request help. Nurses providing such care should be knowledgeable about rehabilitative strategies and ways of encouraging patients to carry out these activities for themselves. In this case, doing these activities for the patient would undermine the plan and might reduce the likelihood of the care outcome being achieved. The nurse giving care might, however, also need to assess the patient and decide whether the patient was indeed too tired to undertake these activities for him- or herself.

Alternatively, if the patient were receiving palliative care, it might be considered appropriate for the nurse to wash or feed the patient if the patient requested this as a greater emphasis might be placed on quality of life as perceived by the patient. It follows that, although the actions and goals of care can be clearly specified in the care plan, the nurse providing the care may need to negotiate the care plan in accordance with the patient's wishes or energy levels at the time that care is given. As Martha Rogers' (1980) work has illustrated, recognising, monitoring and responding to the energy level of the patient is a core nursing function that can simultaneously be affected by the energy level of the nurse.

In discussing the issue of unqualified staff working with primary nursing, Manthey (1991) suggests that health care assistants work in partnership with registered nurses, taking the same shifts and working with the same caseload of patients. This prevents the need for unqualified staff to negotiate the care plan in the absence of the qualified nurse and thus perpetuates the assumption that unqualified nurses do not take care decisions but only carry out delegated tasks, as described by Batey and Lewis (1982) above.

In practice, nursing is characterised by considerable discontinuity and disruption in the team providing care. The ideal situation described by Manthey can be severely compromised by changes in nursing personnel and by the rapid movement of patients from ward to ward or unit to unit (Procter, 1995; Close and Procter, 1999). The rapid movement of patients through wards and units can be reinforced by contemporary management information systems, described earlier, which focus on processing rather than resolving patient care problems.

McKenna (1995) cites evidence indicating that, during the period 1991–92, the number of qualified nurses reduced by 21 per cent in general nursing, 33 per cent in elderly care nursing, 24 per cent in mental health nursing and 17 per cent in learning disabilities nursing in the NHS in England and Wales. In 1993, there was a 21 per cent increase in the number of unqualified nurses employed. A rapid change such as this in the composition of the nursing workforce disrupts continuity of care and undermines the development of shared working practices in the provision of 24-hour care for patients by both qualified and unqualified nurses.

Both Alaszewski (1977) and Procter (1989a) have demonstrated how transience and discontinuity in the nursing workforce give rise to the implementation of care according to ward routines. The more mobile the workforce is between units and wards within the hospital and between hospitals, the more important it is that these routines are shared across all the units and wards through which staff are circulating. This is essential in order to ensure that staff can be fully utilised within the areas to which they have been allocated. Wards implementing care very differently could not utilise these staff and, in a situation of discontinuity and transience, would be unable to provide effective care. In such circumstances, they would be forced to conform to the routine in order to make effective use of transient staff.

Routinised care has traditionally been linked to task-orientated care governed by rules and procedures (Rodgers, 1995), as associated with care-as-duty. Even within primary nursing, the need to provide 24-hour care requires some form of teamworking between nursing staff, even if the overall responsibility for care is located with one individual. While considerable enthusiasm has been expressed for primary nursing (Pearson, 1988; Rodgers, 1995), it is important not to become complacent about the potential of primary nursing to overcome the problems identified with team- or task-orientated nursing (Berry and Metcalf, 1986).

In discussing professional accountability in nursing, it is important to recognise that, while the quality of nursing care is fundamentally dependent on the quality of decision making by the individual care giver, the individual care giver cannot at the same time be responsible for care over a 24-hour period. Instead, responsibility is shared between each of the care givers such that the outcome cannot be attributed to any one individual (Kitson, 1997). It follows that quality care in nursing requires an environment in which teamwork is supported, standards of care are shared and developed, and the nursing team is not constantly disrupted by an influx of transient workers. This has implications not only for the management of the existing workforce, but also for the development of educational curricula in nursing. Short clinical placements that rotate students through an increasing number of clinical environments are likely to have an adverse effect on quality of care by disrupting the stability and development of nursing teams. This suggests the need to monitor nursing team stability as an indicator of the quality of the environment within which nursing is expected to perform.

Accountability in community nursing

The problems of accountability in nursing described above derive from an analysis of hospital nursing. Community nursing provides another context in which the issues of accountability can be analysed. Community nursing has traditionally been characterised by a much higher proportion of qualified staff and has traditionally had a flatter hierarchy than hospital nursing (NHSME, 1992).

In a study of community nursing, Griffiths and Luker (1994) found that nurses were expected to cover for each other in the absence of a colleague. There was, however, a reluctance on the part of the nurse to interfere with a colleague's care plan or to offer an opinion or nursing input with which their colleague might not agree. Furthermore, nurses appeared to be reluctant to commit the resources of a colleague's time by making suggestions for care. This was explained by a lack of knowledge about the colleague's other commitments and by the fact that doing things differently might set a precedent with the patient with which the patient's own nurse would be unable to comply.

Griffiths and Luker point out how the reluctance to comment on or discuss a colleague's care plan militates against peer review and the maintenance of good standards of practice. They go on to suggest that this strategy is not restricted to nursing but is a general characteristic found in many professions (Friedson, 1970). The authors conclude by proposing the emergence of organisational rules that develop to enable the smooth running of the team. These rules do not, however, necessarily promote peer scrutiny or patient choice by indicating alternative approaches to care and allowing patients to decide on their preferred option. As Griffiths and Luker point out, 'mechanisms for discerning moral issues, patterns of communication, self-scrutiny and conflict resolution are substantially under-developed at the present time' (p. 1044).

Understanding the role of nursing routines in determining care outcomes

The existence of nursing routines and organisational rules to arbitrate between the needs of different patients and to maintain the authority of the nurse confounds the principles of individualised care and accountability advocated by primary nursing. However, as Melia (1995) points out, the devolution of decision making and budgets to wards and units serves to highlight the real dilemma in nursing between providing the best care for an individual patient and the best care for the patient/client group as a whole. A key part of the accountability of nursing is managing resources to produce the best balance between these two opposing demands.

Decisions on prioritisation are frequently embedded in nursing routines and organisational rules (Graham, 1984; Procter, 1989a; Griffiths and Luker, 1994) that govern the allocation of care resources and give rise to particular care outcomes as a consequence of adherence to these rules. In such circumstances, it becomes important for nursing to acknowledge the shared aspects of working practices and to examine the implicit rules embedded in these practices for their impact on the quality of patient care and on patient care outcome.

Conclusion

The generalised concern about escalating health care costs in Western societies dominates health policy, health care planning and management. Given the changing demographic and epidemiological profile of these countries, there is a need to promote the self-care efficacy of patients and their carers. This requires the provision of realistic information, the development of long-term therapeutic relationships, a shared understanding of the meaning of the illness and the health beliefs of the patient and family, and the reduction of the social exclusion of people experiencing enduring physical and/or mental illness and disability.

Health care policy is increasingly recognising the importance of developing patient-centred services and relocating resources to meet the expressed needs of patients and their families (Borst-Eilers, 1997). From a policy perspective, a concern for effective functioning and self-efficacy among patients derives from the need to reduce the spiralling demand for hospital services, which still represents the biggest single cost to health care. The prevalent ideology adopted by planners is, however, dominated by biomedical models of health derived from physical sciences, which assumes that all illness is derived from physical causes and is amenable to physical cures bought about through technological solutions. The structures and organisations of health care reflect this assumption, giving rise to selective policies of provision, even though the epidemiological and demographic evidence disputes it and highlights the value of more universal approaches.

The analysis presented in this chapter raises very real concerns about whether technological solutions to health care management (as depicted by Spurgeon, 1993) are going to enable health services to address the fundamental problems arising from the long-term disability and the ageing of the population that confront most Western societies. While they might permit the cost of health care to be accurately located in cost centres and thus promote sound budgeting practice, this might be achieved at the expense of addressing the fundamental needs of the patients.

If the work of nurses that focuses on the long-term development and adaptation of the patient to the illness and the management of the illness is marginalised and excluded from health care, this is likely in itself to produce spiralling costs. These costs arise from the increasing and unpredictable demands on health service resources made by patients suffering from long-term disabilities but treated, on each occasion, as an acute and discrete illness episode or event, unrelated in social, psychological, emotional and frequently physical terms to any previous illness episode.

If we are to address contemporary health care needs, health care planners and health economists have to learn to appreciate new definitions and ideologies of health, as outlined in Chapter 2, in order to understand the potential contribution that nursing and other health care professions could make to health care. This chapter has demonstrated that many of the goals of current health care policies, including the containment of spiralling costs and the development of patient-centred services, require the work ascribed to nurses to form a crucial element of the health care agenda. The language of nursing work, however, with its emphasis on the long-term development of the patient, which requires the social, psychological and emotional needs of the patient to be addressed during the course of care giving, is severely disruptive to contemporary health care routines. As this and the previous chapter demonstrate, current management practice emphasises the importance of these routines by costing them and incorporating them into ever more sophisticated management systems. These systems displace nursing work to the margins of health service practice and render it invisible within the service.

Hence, it follows that any dialogue between nurses and health service planners and managers is bound to be problematic as each is dealing with a different agenda arising from different premises about the nature of health care and the provision of appropriate services. As this chapter has demonstrated, however, the concerns of health service planners and managers to reduce spiralling costs can be achieved through the work of nurses to facilitate patient self-efficacy by improving the quality of life of patients and the health outcomes of patients and their families.

It would appear that the ultimate goals of nurses, planners and managers in relation to patient outcome are the same. What prevents them communicating effectively is the lack of shared understanding of the processes by which this can be achieved. The evidence presented in this chapter indicates that, by addressing the emotional, social and psychological as well as physical needs of patients, the processes associated with nursing work are likely to be more effective in achieving health service goals than is concentrating on technical efficiency alone. The problem for nurses, planners, and health service managers is that addressing the holistic needs of patients requires a restructuring of service provision in order to promote a holistic and universal service response. Achieving this runs contrary to most of the deep-seated beliefs about efficiency and cost-effectiveness that currently dominate health service thinking and simultaneously undermine the potential achievements of nursing in promoting health.

Chapter 9

Concluding Remarks

This book has argued the case for recognising the importance of caring work to health promotion and health maintenance in the context of illness regardless of who performs this work and where it is carried out. The book has chronicled the marginalisation of caring work from formal organisational structures, policy debates and reward systems. It has highlighted the importance of new ways of working to achieve caring work. These include a recognition of the importance of reciprocity between carers, including formal and informal carers; of undertaking seemingly menial and trivial tasks such as doing the ironing while simultaneously supporting families dealing with life and death situations; of recognising the features of caring work, including dependency, emotional labour, intimacy, nurturing and vulnerability, as being central to work for health; and of developing organisational forms and structures designed to support caring practices that address these issues.

Health care reforms in the UK are currently focusing on reconfiguring the boundaries between services. They are not, however, addressing the central boundary between formal and informal care or identifying the working practices and institutional supports required to bring about effective caring wherever caring is practised. Caring work has traditionally been located in the privatised sphere of the family. Here, it has been depoliticised and marginalised from mainstream organisational structures that confer power, prestige, status and rewards. There is, however, a growing body of evidence that testifies to the damage to health deriving from a failure to care, whether this failure is located in the family or arises out of the practice of paid carers.

The centrality of caring work to health is illustrated by Donaldson and Donaldson (1993) in a review of public health practice. They suggest that the potential to improve health is enormous if ways can be found by which to modify risk factors on a population scale and help people to adopt and sustain healthy lifestyles. They state:

> Much of the key to success lies in shaping the behaviour and values of children and young people. It lies in enabling them to lay the foundations for a life which will achieve the maximum of the biological span and in which most of those years will be characterised by health rather than illness, chronic disease or disability. If these challenges can be met, as the world moves towards the next millennium, then the scale of public health achievement will be as great as the historical discoveries which transformed the health landscape of the past. (Donaldson and Donaldson, 1993, p. 175)

The work of Donaldson and Donaldson (1993) indicates that healthy behaviour over time is incorporated into the patterns and routines of daily living that circumscribe and engulf our daily lives, in diet, in exercise, in leisure and in the ability and opportunity to socialise. This book argues that nurses, in their everyday practice, oversee and substitute for one form of family care, the tending care associated with supporting and maintaining activities of daily living over a 24-hour period. In their work, nurses regularly breach the boundaries between formal and informal family care. The way in which they do this, and the knowledge to be gained from studying both the caring practices of families and the practices of nurses working at the interface between formal and informal care, is central to understanding how care promotes health, when care fails and how failures in care can be prevented.

The way forward

Reintegrating caring work into mainstream political and economic structures of society requires:

- The recognition of a need for care independent of a need for biomedical intervention so that admission to expensive (in terms of cost per bed per day) technical hospital facilities is restricted to those in need of this type of intervention and those for whom there is evidence that it is clinically effective. Hospital services are currently available on demand (through A&E services), free at the point of access and non-stigmatising. Reducing the demand for expensive hospital services requires that these characteristics be replicated for those who simply require access to care rather than medical intervention, otherwise health service professionals are under pressure to interpret a need for care as a biomedical need for technical intervention in order for patients and carers to gain access to the level of care available in hospital settings.

- The impact of nursing theories and models, and the findings from nursing research, need to be tested to evaluate their impact on health care outcomes for patients, families and communities. This might start to address the question 'How many nurses do we need?' by identifying whether providing differing levels and skill mix in nursing for different population groups can partially compensate for inequality in health care outcomes.

- The development of organisational structures and practices that support continuity of care and, where possible, the nurse carer across primary, secondary and tertiary sectors and over time. This is necessary in order accurately to assess care needs and provide a care input appropriate to managing fluctuating health and disease trajectories.

- There is a need to develop an economics of caring alongside an economics of health so that the full costs, including opportunity costs, of caring activities can be calculated and integrated into mainstream economic analysis. Opportunity costs are associated with opportunities forgone by informal carers as well as the opportunities lost when nursing care focuses on managing the throughput of patients, for example the readmission of patients to hospital, rather than addressing and resolving the care needs that may well be giving rise to the readmission.

- There is a need for health care practitioners to recognise that, if patients are to collaborate equally with them in promoting and maintaining health, maintaining and enhancing the moral integrity and identity of the person receiving care is central to the interaction.

- A recognition that, for each of us, caring distinguishes what we feel passionate about. Understanding what people, including health care professionals, care about indicates where energy is located in the system and how priorities will be determined in practice rather than in strategies. This type of understanding is fundamental to effecting change and promoting clinical effectiveness.

Service planning is currently linked to biomedical measures such as mortality and morbidity. In the context of the increasing prevalence of chronic disease described in Chapter 3, such measures fail accurately to reflect health care need because they do not provide information on factors such as the personal significance, meaning and interpretation of symptoms; self-management and coping strategies; anxiety, compliance and motivation; and the experience of living with the illness within the family unit. Addressing these issues requires:

- Integrating evidence derived from the daily life experiences of patients, carers and the communities in which they live and work with evidence from professional sources of knowledge in order to produce integrated and meaningful services for both patients and professionals.

- Reducing inequality in access to service provision and providing targeted, selective services within a universal and accessible model of provision embedded in the culture of local communities.

- The provision of clinically effective, selective, targeted interventions arising from an understanding, shared between the patient, the patient's carer and the professional, of the individual needs of the patient and/or carer within a universal framework of provision.

- The development of an integrated whole-system approach to service provision that will foster social integration for patients and their carers. This will involve patient/carer representation, the voluntary sector, the business sector and local authority services (for example, social services, leisure, transport, housing and town planning) working alongside health service interventions.

- The development of integrated data sets encompassing psychosocial indicators (psychosocial adjustment, sense of coherence, quality of life and social support networks) and demographic data as well as mortality and morbidity data.

This is the agenda to which nursing can make a substantial contribution. Nursing theories and knowledge derived from social science perspectives, about individualised, patient-centred care and the formal and informal caring needs of patients, means that nursing work complements biomedical knowledge derived from the physical sciences. The phenomenological approach to research and evidence that characterises nursing provides an important element of the knowledge required to realise the vision set out by Donaldson and Donaldson (1993) above.

In advocating the reintegration of caring work into the mainstream political and economic structure of society, it is recognised that the frequently voiced concern with professional encroachment and the deskilling of family carers is very real and fully justified. This concern will materialise if the integrity of caring work is not fully understood and appreciated by those who are charged with its provision. In particular, providers need to be aware of the ways in which caring work contravenes the traditional understanding of bureaucracies, professionalisation and hierarchical forms of control. Providers need to appreciate the importance of reciprocity between carers, of control over time, of integrating seemingly trivial tasks with complex questions of life and death, abuse and support, dependency and inter-dependency.

If these features of caring work, and others not yet identified, are not understood and supported by organisations providing health and social care, and if the importance of these features for effective caring within families is not studied and where appropriate supported, the professionalisation of caring could lead to the eradication of caring behaviours from society. Alternatively, if the role of caring in promoting health and well-being is studied, and appropriate support is provided to those who find themselves in a caring situation, caring activities may be transformed from an association with burden and drudgery to an interpretation of caring as a life-enhancing and satisfying human and humane activity.

References

Abel-Smith, B. (1994) *Introduction to Health Policy, Planning and Financing*. London, Longman.

Abrams, P. (1980) 'Social change, social networks and neighbourhood care'. *Social Work Service* (22nd February): 12–23.

Agency for Health Care Policy and Research (1992) *Urinary Incontinence in Adults: Clinical Practice Guidelines*. Washington, DC, Public Health Services, US Department of Health and Human Services.

Aggleton, P. J. and Chalmers, H. (1986) *Nursing Models and the Nursing Process*. Basingstoke, Macmillan.

Alaszewski, A. M. (1977) 'Suggestions for the reorganisation of nurse training and improvement of patient care in a hospital for the mentally handicapped'. *Journal of Advanced Nursing* 2: 461–77.

Anthony, P. D. (1977) *The Ideology of Work*. London, Tavistock.

Antonovsky, A. (1993) 'The structure and properties of the sense of coherence scale'. *Social Science and Medicine* 36(6): 725–33.

Antonovsky, A. (1996) 'The salutogenic model as a theory to guide health promotion'. *Health Promotion International* 11(1): 11–18.

Armstrong, D. (1984) 'The patient's view'. *Social Science and Medicine* 18: 737–44.

Armstrong, D. (1987) 'Theoretical tensions in biopsychosocial medicine'. *Social Science and Medicine* 25: 1213–18.

Arnold, J. and Breen, L. J. (1998) 'Images of health', in Gorin, S. S. and Arnold, J. (eds) *Health Promotion Handbook*. St Louis, Mosby, pp. 3–13.

Ashton, J. (ed.) (1992) *Healthy Cities*. Milton Keynes, Open University Press.

Ashton, J. and Seymour, H. (1988) *The New Public Health. The Liverpool Experience*. Buckingham, Open University Press.

Atkins, P. J. (1992) 'White poison? The social consequences of milk consumption in London 1850–1939'. *Social History of Medicine* 5(2): 207–27.

Audit Commission (1991) *The Virtue of Patients: Making Best Use of Ward Nursing Resources*. HMSO, London.

Audit Commission (1992) *Community Care: Managing the Cascade of Change*. HMSO, London.

Baker, D. E. (1983) '"Care" in the geriatric ward: an account of two styles of nursing', in Wilson-Barnett, J. (ed.) *Nursing Research: Ten Case Studies*. Chichester, Wiley, pp. 101–17.

Baldwin, S. and Twigg, J. (1991) 'Women and community care – reflections on a debate', in Maclean, M. and Groves, D. (eds) *Women's Issues in Social Policy*. London, Routledge, pp. 117–35.

Barker, D. (1992) *Fetal and Infant Origins of Disease in Adult Life*. London, BMA.

Barnard, K. A. (1977) 'Promises, patients and politics: the conflicts of the NHS', in Barnard, K. A. and Lee, K. (eds) *Conflicts in the National Health Service*. London, Croom Helm, pp. 13–25.

Barr, A. (1967) *Measurement of Nursing Care*. Oxford, Oxford Regional Hospital Board.

Bartley, M., Blane, D. and Montgomery, S. (1997) 'Health and the life course: why safety nets matter'. *British Medical Journal* **314**: 1194–6.

Batey, M. V. and Lewis, F. M. (1982) 'Clarifying autonomy and accountability in the nursing service'. *Journal of Nursing Administration* **12**(9): 13–18.

Bebbington, A. (1991) 'The expectation of life without disability in England and Wales: 1976–88'. *Population Trends* **66**: 26–9.

Benner, P. (1997) *From Novice to Expert: Experiential Learning in Caring for Chronic Illness*. Empowerment of the Chronically Ill: A Challenge for Nursing. Amsterdam, paper presented at 2nd European Nursing Congress.

Benner, P. and Wrubel, J. (1989) *The Primacy of Caring: Stress and Coping in Health and Illness*. Menlo Park, CA, Addison-Wesley.

Berry, A. J. and Metcalf, C. L. (1986) 'Paradigms and practices: the organisation and delivery of nursing care'. *Journal of Advanced Nursing* **11**(5): 589–97.

Bjork, I. T. (1995) 'Neglected conflicts in the discipline of nursing: perceptions of the importance and value of practical skills'. *Journal of Advanced Nursing* **22**: 6–12.

Blane, D., Brunner, E. and Wilkinson, R. (eds) (1996) *Health and Social Organisation*. London, Routledge.

Blaxter, M. (1981) *The Health of the Children. A Review of Research on the Place of Health in the Cycle of Disadvantage*. London, Heinemann.

Blaxter, M. (1995) 'What is health?', in Davey, B. G. and Seale, A. (eds) *Health and Disease: A Reader*. Buckingham, Open University Press, pp. 26–32.

Boeije, H. R., van den Dungen A. W. L., Pool, A., Grypdonck, M. H. F. and van Lieshout, P. A. H. (1997) *Future Scenarios for Nursing in the Netherlands*. Empowerment of the Chronically Ill: A Challenge for Nursing. Amsterdam, paper presented at 2nd European Nursing Congress.

Bond, S. and Thomas, L. (1991) 'Issues in measuring outcomes of nursing'. *Journal of Advanced Nursing* **16**: 52–63.

Borst-Eilers, E. (1997) *Government Policy on the Chronically Ill*. Empowerment of the Chronically Ill: A Challenge for Nursing. Amsterdam, paper presented at 2nd European Nursing Congress.

Bottorff, J. (1997) *Palliative Care: Autonomy within Dependency*. Empowerment of the Chronically Ill: A Challenge for Nursing. Amsterdam, paper presented at 2nd European Nursing Congress.

Bowlby, J. (1969) *Attachment and Loss*. Vol. 1: *Attachment*. London, Hogarth.

Bowlby, J. (1973) *Attachment and Loss* Vol. 2: *Separation: Anxiety and Anger*. London, Hogarth.

Bowlby, J. (1980) *Attachment and Loss*. Vol. 3: *Sadness and Depression*. London, Hogarth.

Bowling, A. (1997) *Research Methods in Health Investigating Health and Health Services*. Buckingham, Open University Press.

Boyle, J.S and Andrews, M.M. (1989) *Transcultural Concepts in Nursing Care*. Glenview, Scott Foresman/Little.

Bradshaw, J. (1972) 'A taxonomy of social need', in McLachlan, G. (ed.) *Problems and Progress in Medical Care*. Oxford, Nuffield Provincial Hospital Trust, pp. 69–82.

Bradshaw, J. R. (1994) 'A conceptualisation and measurement of need: a social policy perspective', in Popay, J. and Williams, G. (eds) *Researching the People's Health*. London, Routledge, pp. 45–57.

Branckaerts, J. and Richardson, A. (1992) 'Self-help groups: their impact and potential', in Kaplun, A. (ed.) *Health Promotion and Chronic Illness: Discovering a New Quality of Life*. Copenhagen, WHO Regional Office for Europe, pp. 363–7.

Browne, G., Roberts, J., Bryne, C. and Gafni, A. (1994) 'The cost of poor adjustment to chronic illness: lessons from three studies'. *Health and Social Care* 2: 85–93.

Brykczynska, G. (1992) 'Caring – a dying art?', in Jolley, M. and Brykczynska, G. (eds) *Nursing Care: The Challenge to Change*. London, Edward Arnold, pp. 1–45.

Brykczynska, G. (1997) 'A brief overview of the epistimology of caring', in Byrkczynska, G. (ed.) *Caring: The Compassion and Wisdom of Nursing*. London, Arnold, pp. 1–9.

Budd, S. (1994) 'Transference revisited', in Budd, S. and Sharma, U. (eds) *The Healing Bond: The Patient–Practitioner Relationship and Therapeutic Responsibility*. London, Routledge, pp. 153–70.

Bulmer, M. (1987) *The Social Basis of Community Care*. London, Allen & Unwin.

Bunting, S. (1993) *Rosemarie Parse: Theory of Human Becoming*. London, Sage.

Burckhardt, C. S. (1987) 'Coping strategies of the chronically ill'. *Nursing Clinics of North America* 22(3): 543–9.

Burnard, P. (1997) 'Why care? Ethical and spiritual issues in caring in nursing', in Brykczynska, G. (ed.) *Caring: The Compassion and Wisdom of Nursing*. London, Arnold, pp. 32–44.

Callery, P. (1997) 'Maternal knowledge and professional knowledge: co-operation and conflict in the care of sick children'. *International Journal of Nursing Studies* 34(1): 27–34.

Campbell, B. (1993) *Goliath Britain's Dangerous Places*. London, Methuen.

Capra, F. (1982) *The Turning Point: Science, Society and the Rising Culture*. London, Fontana.

Carpenter, M. (1993) 'The subordination of nurses in health care: towards a social divisions approach', in Riska, E. and Wegar, K. (eds) *Gender, Work and Medicine: Women and the Medical Division of Labour*. London, Sage, pp. 95–130.

Carr-Hill, R. A. and Jenkins-Clarke, S. (1995) 'Measurement systems in principle and in practice: the example of nursing workload'. *Journal of Advanced Nursing* 22: 221–5.

Casey, A. (1995) 'Partnership nursing: influences on involvement of informal carers'. *Journal of Advanced Nursing* 22: 1058–62.

Charlton, J. (1997) 'Trends in all-cause mortality 1841–1994', in Charlton, J. and Murphy, M. (eds) *The Health of Adult Britain 1841–1994*. London, Office for National Statistics, Vol. 1, pp. 17–29.

Charlton, D. and Murphy, M. (eds) (1997a) *Adult Health: Historical Aspects 1850–1980*. London, HMSO.

Charlton, J. and Murphy, M. (1997b) *The Health of Adult Britain 1841–1994*. London, Office for National Statistics.

Charlton, J., Fraser, P. and Murphy, M. (1997) 'Medical advances and iatrogensis', in Charlton, J. and Murphy, M. (eds) *The Health of Adult Britain 1841–1994*. London, Office for National Statistics, 1: 217–30.

Cheater, F. M. (1991) 'Attitudes towards incontinence'. *Nursing Standard* 5(26): 23–7.

Chief Medical Officer (1998) *Chief Medical Officer's Project to Strengthen the Public Health Function: Report of Emerging Findings*. London, DoH, (microfiche – interlibrary loan).

Clarke, A. (1996) 'Why are we trying to reduce length of stay? Evaluation of the costs and benefits of reducing time in hospital must start from the objectives that govern the change'. *Quality in Health Care* 5: 172–9.

Close, H. and Procter, S. (1999) 'Coping strategies used by hospitalized stroke patients: implications for continuity and management of care'. *Journal of Advanced Nursing* **29**(1): 138–44.

Coates, V. E and Boore, J. P. R. (1996) 'Knowledge and diabetes self-management'. *Patient Education and Counseling* **29**: 98–108.

Cochrane, A. L., St Ledger, A. S. and Moore, F. (1978) 'Health service "input" and mortality "output" in developed countries'. *Journal of Epidemiology and Community Health* **32**: 200–5.

Connelly, C. E. (1987) 'Self-care and the chronically ill patient'. *Nursing Clinics of North America* **22**(3): 621–3.

Council of Europe (1986) *Organisation of Prevention in Primary Care*. Strasbourg, Council of Europe.

Coveney, I. (1983) 'Belt, buckle, badge'. *Nursing Times* **79**(48): 72.

Coyne, J. C. (1995) 'Intervention in close relationhips to improve coping with illness', in Lyons, R. F., Sullivan, M. J. L. and Ritvo, P. G. (eds) *Relationships in Chronic Illness and Disability*. London, Sage, pp. 96–122.

Croom, S. (1996) An exploration of control in child and adolescent psychiatric nursing practice: analysis and meta-analysis. Unpublished Msc thesis, University of Northumbria, Newcastle.

Davies, C. (1992) 'Gender, history and management style in nursing: towards a theoretical synthesis', in Savage, M. and Witz, A. (eds) *Gender and Bureaucracy*. Oxford, Blackwell, pp. 229–52.

Davies, C. (1995) *Gender and the Professional Predicament in Nursing*. Buckingham, Open University Press.

Davies, J. (1995) 'A study of family networks and relationships in community midwifery', in Reed, J. and Procter, S. (eds) *Practitioner Research in Health Care: The Inside Story*. London, Chapman & Hall, pp. 130–46.

Department of Health (1996a) *Primary Care: Delivering the Future*. London, HMSO.

Department of Health (1996b) *The National Health Service: A Service with Ambitions*. London, HMSO.

Department of Health (1997) *On the State of Public Health: the Annual Report of the Clinical Medical Officer of the Department of Health*. London, HMSO.

Department of Health (1998a) *Partnership in Action: New Opportunities for Joint Working between Health and Social Services*. London, DoH.

Department of Health (1998b) *Healthy Living Centres: Report of a Seminar Held on 2 April 1998*. London, DoH.

Department of Health (1998c) *The New NHS: Modern and Dependable Executive Summary*. London, HMSO.

Department of Health (1998d) *Information for Health*. London, HMSO.

Department of Health (1999) *Making a Difference: Strengthening the Nursing, Midwifery and Health Visiting Contribution to Health and Healthcare*. London, HMSO.

Department of Health and Social Security (1968) *Report of the Committee on Local Authority and Allied Personnel Social Services*. [Seebohm Report] London, HMSO.

Department of Health and Social Security (1982a) *Mix and Match: A Review of Nursing Skill Mix*. London, HMSO.

Department of Health and Social Security (1982b) *Nurse Manpower: Maintaining the Balance*. London.

Department of Health and Social Security (1983) *Nurse Manpower: Planning Approaches and Techniques.* London, HMSO.

Department of Social Services (1988) *Report of the Committee of Inquiry into the Future Development of the Public Health Function in England and Wales.* [Acheson Report] London, HMSO.

Dickinson, S. (1982) 'The nursing process and the professional status of nursing'. *Nursing Times* **78**(16): 61–4.

Donaldson, C. and Gerard, K. (1993) *Economics of Health Care: Financing the Visible Hand.* Basingstoke, Macmillan.

Donaldson, R. J. and Donaldson, L. J. (1993) *Essential Public Health Medicine.* London, Kluwer Academic Press.

Douglas, M. (1994) 'The construction of the physician: a cultural approach to medical fashions', in Budd, S. and Sharma, U. (eds) *The Healing Bond: The Patient–Practitioner Relationship and Therapeutic Responsibility.* London, Routledge, pp. 23–40.

Doyal, L. and Gough, I. (1991) *A Theory of Human Need.* Basingstoke, Macmillan.

Dunlop, M. J. (1986) 'Is a science of caring possible?' *Journal of Advanced Nursing* **11**: 661–70.

English National Board for Nursing, Midwifery and Health Visiting (1999) 'Preparation for the developing role of the community children's nurse'. *Researching Professional Education* – Research Report Series No. 11. London, ENB.

Ersser, S. (1991) 'A search for the therapeutic dimensions of nurse–patient interaction', in McMahon, R. and Pearson, A. (eds) *Nursing as Therapy.* London, Chapman & Hall, pp. 43–84.

Essen, J. and Wedge, P. (1982) *Continuities in Childhood Disadvantage.* London, Heinemann.

Farquhar, M. (1995) 'Definitions of quality of life: a taxonomy'. *Journal of Advanced Nursing* **22**: 502–8.

Farsides, C. (1994) Autonomy, responsibility and midwifery', in Budd, S. and Sharma, U. (eds) *The Healing Bond: The Patient–Practitioner Relationship and Therapeutic Responsibility.* London, Routledge, pp. 42–62.

Fawcett, J. (1989) *Analysis and Evaluation of Conceptual Models in Nursing.* Philadelphia, F. A. Davis.

Finch, J. (1984) 'Community care: developing non-sexist alternatives'. *Critical Social Policy* **9**: 6–18.

Flaskerud, J. H. and Winslow, B. J. (1998) 'Conceptualising vulnerable populations health related research'. *Nursing Research* **47**(2): 69–77.

Freidson, E. (1970) *Professional Dominance: The Social Structure of Medical Care.* Chicago, Aldine.

Fretwell, J. E. (1982) *Ward Teaching and Learning.* London, RCN.

Frey, M. A. (1995) *Advancing King's System Framework and Theory of Nursing.* London, Sage.

Fries, J. (1980) 'Aging, natural death and the compression of morbidity'. *New England Journal of Medicine* **303**: 130–5.

Froland, C. (1980) 'Formal and informal care: discontinuities on a continuum'. *Social Service Review* **54**(4): 572–87.

Gault, A. R. (1982) 'The Aberdeen formula as an illustration of the difficulty of determining nursing requirements'. *International Journal of Nursing Studies* **19**(2): 61–77.

Gilligan, C. (1982) *In a Different Voice: Psychological Theory and Women's Development.* Harvard, Harvard University Press.

Goddard, H. A. (1953) *The Work of Nurses in General Hospital Wards. Report of a Job Analysis.* London, Nuffield Provincial Hospital Trusts.

Gould, C. C. (1984) 'Private rights and public virtues: women, the family, and democracy', in Gould, C. C. (ed.) *Beyond Domination: New Perspectives on Women and Philosophy.* Totowa, NJ, Rowman & Allanheld, pp. 3–18.

Gould, C. (1996) 'Multiple partnership in the community'. *Paediatric Nursing* **8**(8): 27–31.

Graham, H. (1984) *Women, Health and the Family.* London, Harvester Wheatsheaf.

Griffiths, J. M. and Luker, K. A. (1994) 'Intraprofessional teamwork in district nursing: in whose interest?' *Journal of Advanced Nursing* **20**: 1038–45.

Grimshaw, J. M. and Russell, I. T. (1993) 'Achieving health gain through clinical guidelines. 1: Developing scientifically valid guidelines'. *Quality in Health Care* **2**: 243–8.

Grossman, M. (1972) *The Demand for Health: A Theoretical and Empirical Investigation.* New York, National Bureau of Economic Research.

Grundy, E. (1997) 'The health and health care of older adults in England and Wales, 1841–1994', in Charlton, J. and Murphy, M. (eds) *The Health of Adult Britain 1841–1994.* London, Office for National Statistics, Vol. 2, pp. 182–203.

Gull, H. J. (1987) 'The chronically ill patient's adaptation to hospitalization'. *Nursing Clinics of North America* **22**(3): 593–601.

Hardie, M. (1978) 'Auxiliaries: who needs them? A case study in nursing', in Hardie, M. and Hockey, L. (eds) *Nursing Auxiliaries in Health Care.* London, Croom Helm, pp. 42–51.

Health Advisory Service (1995) *The Commissioning Role and Management of Child and Adolescent Mental Health Services. Together We Stand.* NHS Health Advisory Thematic Review. London, Stationery Office.

Held, V. (1993) *Feminist Morality: Transforming Culture, Society and Politics.* Chicago, University of Chicago Press.

Holzt, K. and Wilson, P. D. (1988) 'The prevalence of female urinary incontinence and reasons for not seeking treatment'. *New Zealand Medical Journal* **101**: 756–8.

Houghton, A., Bowling, A., Clarke, K. D., Hopkins, A. P. and Jones, I. (1996) 'Does a dedicated discharge coordinator improve the quality of hospital discharge'. *Quality in Health Care* **5**(2): 89–96.

Hurst, K. (1993) *Nurse Workforce Planning.* Harrow, Longman.

James, A. (1994) *Managing to Care: Public Service and the Market.* London, Longman.

James, N. (1992) 'Care=organisation+physical labour+emotional labour'. *Sociology of Health and Illness* **14**(4): 489–509.

Jenkins-Clarke, S. (1992) *Measuring Nursing Workload: A Cautionary Tale.* York, Centre for Health Economics Health Economics Consortium, University of York.

Johnson, D. E. (1980) 'The behavioural system model for nursing', in Riehl, J. P. and Roy, C. (eds) *Conceptual Models for Nursing Practice.* New York, Appleton-Century-Crofts, (2nd edn), pp. 207–16.

Joshi, H. (1991) 'Sex and motherhood as handicaps in the labour market', in Maclean, M. and Groves, D. (eds) *Womens Issues in Social Policy.* London, Routledge, pp. 179–93.

Kaplun, A. (ed.) (1992) *Health Promotion and Chronic Illness.* Copenhagen, WHO Regional Office for Europe.

Kelly, M. P. and May, D. (1982) 'Good and bad patients: a review of the literature and a theoretical critique', *Journal of Advanced Nursing* 7: 147–56.

Keyzer, D. (1992) 'Nursing policy, the supply and demand for nurses: towards a clinical career structure for nurses', in Robinson, J. Gray, A. and Elkan, R. (eds) *Policy Issues in Nursing*. Milton Keynes, Open University Press, pp. 112–19.

Kitson, A. (1987) 'A comparative analysis of lay-caring and professional (nursing) caring relationships'. *International Journal of Nursing Studies* 24(2): 155–65.

Kitson, A. (1993) 'Formalising concepts related to nursing and caring', in Kitson, A. (ed.) *Nursing Art and Science*. London, Chapman & Hall, pp. 25–47.

Kitson, A. (1997) 'Using evidence to demonstrate the value of nursing'. *Nursing Standard* 11(28): 34–9.

Kitson, A. (1999a) 'The essence of nursing part i'. *Nursing Standard* 13(23): 42–6.

Kitson, A. (1999b) 'The essence of nursing part ii'. *Nursing Standard* 13(24): 34–6.

Knight, R. and Procter, S. (1999) 'Implementation of clinical guidelines for female urinary incontinence: a comparative analysis of organizational structures and service delivery'. *Health and Social Care in the Community* 7(4): 239–310.

Knight, R., Procter, S., Watson, B., Dryden, J. and Lawson, C. (1999) Evidence based practice: clinical guidelines and the management of female urinary incontinence. Unpublished Report, NHSE Northern and Yorkshire.

Kratz, C. R. (1979) *The Nursing Process*. London, Baillière Tindall.

Kuhse, H. (1997) *Caring: Nurses, Women and Ethics*. Oxford, Blackwell.

Lawler, J. (1991) *Behind the Screens: Nursing, Somology and the Problem of the Body*. Edinburgh, Churchill Livingstone.

Lazarus, R. S. (1992) 'Coping with the stress of illness', in Kaplun, A. (ed.) *Health Promotion and Chronic Illness: Discovering a New Quality of Health*. Copenhagen, WHO Regional Office for Europe, pp. 11–31.

Leddy, S. and Pepper, J. M. (1993) *Conceptual Bases of Professional Nursing*. Philadelphia, Lippincott.

Le Grand, J. (1982) *The Struggle of Inequality*. London, Allen & Unwin.

Leininger, M. M. (1988) 'Leininger's theory of nursing: cultural care diversity and universality'. *Nursing Science Quarterly* 1: 152–60.

Lerner, M. (1992) 'Emerging forces in cancer care', in Kaplun, A (ed.) *Health Promotion and Chronic Illness: Discovering a New Quality of Life*. Copenhagen, WHO Regional Office for Europe, pp. 115–39.

Lipsky, M. (1991) 'The paradox of managing discretionary workers in social welfare policy', in Adler, M., Bell, C., Clasen, J. and Sinfield, A. (eds) *The Sociology of Social Security*. Edinburgh, Edinburgh University Press, pp. 212–28.

Litwak, E. and Szelenyi, I. (1969) 'Primary group structures and their functions: kin, neighbours and friends'. *American Sociological Review* 34: 465–81.

Lyons, R. F., Sullivan, M. J. L. and Ritvo, P. G. (1995) *Relationships in Chronic Illness and Disability*. London, Sage.

McCubbin, M. A. and McCubbin, H. I. (1993) 'Families coping with illness: the resiliency model of family stress, adjustment and adaptation', in Danielson, C. B., Hamel-Bissell, B. and Winstead-Fry, P. (eds) *Families, Health and Illness*. St Louis, Mosby, pp. 21–64.

MacDonald, T. H. (1998) *Rethinking Health Promotion*. London, Routledge.

MacGuire, J. M. (1988) 'Dependency matters: an issue in the care of elderly people', in White, R. (ed.) *Political Issues in Nursing Past, Present and Future*. Chichester, Wiley, pp. 71–94.

Mackay, L. (1989) *Nursing a Problem.* Milton Keynes, Open University Press.

McKee, C. (1991) 'Breaking the mould: a humanistic approach to nursing practice', in McMahon, R. and Pearson, A. *Nursing as Therapy.* London, Chapman & Hall, pp. 170–91.

McKee, M., Aiken, L., Rafferty, A. M. and Sochalski, J. (1998) 'Organisational change and quality of health care: an evolving international agenda'. *Quality in Health Care* 7: 37–41.

McKenna, H. (1995) 'Nursing skill mix substitutions and quality of care: an exploration of assumptions from the research literature'. *Journal of Advanced Nursing* 21: 452–9.

McKenna, H. (1997) *Nursing Theories and Models.* London, Routledge.

McKeown, T. (1979) *The Role of Modern Medicine.* Oxford, Blackwell.

McLachlan, G. (1990) *What Price Quality? The NHS in Review.* London, Nuffield Provisional Hospitals Trust.

McMahon, R. (1991) 'Therapeutic nursing: theory, issues and practice', in McMahon, R. and Pearson, A. (eds) *Nursing as Therapy.* London, Chapman & Hall, pp. 1–25.

Manthey, M. (1980) *The Practice of Primary Nursing.* Boston, Blackwell.

Manthey, M. (1991) 'Primary partners'. *Nursing Times* 87(25): 27–8.

Manton, K. (1982) 'Changing concepts of morbidity and mortality in the elderly population'. *Millbank Memorial Fund Quarterly* 60: 133–224.

Marchione, J. (1993) *Margaret Newman: Health as Expanding Consciousness.* London, Sage.

Maslow, A. H. (1987) *Motivation and Personality.* New York, HarperCollins.

May, C. (1995) 'Patient autonomy and the politics of professional relationships'. *Journal of Advanced Nursing* 21: 83–7.

Mayeroff, M. (1972) *On Caring.* New York, Harper & Row.

Maynard, A. (1994) 'Prioritising health care – dreams and reality', in Malek, M. (ed.) *Setting Priorities in Health Care.* Chichester, Wiley, pp. 1–18.

Melia, K. (1995) 'Accountability – the ethical dimension', in Watson, R. (ed.) *Accountability in Nursing Practice.* London, Chapman & Hall, pp. 177–80.

Menzies, I. (1960) *A Case Study in the Functioning of Social Systems as a Defence Against Anxiety.* London, Tavistock.

Miller, A. (1995) *The Drama of Being a Child.* London, Virago.

Milz, H. (1992) '"Healthy ill people": social cynicism or new perspectives?', in Kaplun, A. (ed.) *Health Promotion and Chronic Illness: Discovering a New Quality of Life.* Copenhagen, WHO Regional Office for Europe, pp. 32–9.

Moher, D., Weinberg, A., Hanlon, R. and Runnals, K. (1992) 'Effects of a medical team coordinator on length of hospital stay'. *Canadian Medical Association Journal* 146: 511–15.

Morris, M., Levenback, C., Burke, T. W., Dejesus, Y., Lucas, K. R. and Gersehnson, D. M. (1997) 'An outcomes management program in gynecologic oncology'. *Obstetrics and Gynecology* 89(4): 485–92.

Morse, J. M., Bottorff, J., Neander, W. and Solberg, S. (1991) 'Comparative analysis of conceptualisations and theories of caring'. *Image* 23(2): 119–26.

Moser, K., Goldblatt, P., Fox, J. and Jones, D. (1990) 'Unemployment and mortality', in Goldblatt P. (ed.) *Longitudinal Study: Mortality and Social Organisation.* London, HMSO, pp. 81–97.

National Health Service Management Executive (1992) *The Nursing Skillmix in the District Nursing Service*. London, NHSE Management Executive Value for Money Team, HMSO.

Naylor, M. D. (1990) 'Comprehensive discharge planning for hospitalised elderly: a pilot study'. *Nursing Research* **39**(3): 156–61.

Neidlinger, S. H., Scroggins, K. and Kennedy, L. M. (1987) 'Cost evaluation of discharge planning for hospitalised elderly'. *Nursing Economics* **5**(5): 225–30.

Newby, N. M. (1996) 'Chronic illness and the family life-style'. *Journal of Advanced Nursing* **23**: 786–91.

Newman, S. (1984) 'Anxiety, hospitalisation and surgery', in Fitzpatrick, R., Hinton, J., Newman, S., Scambler, G. and Thompson, J. (eds) *The Experience of Illness*. London, Tavistock, pp. 132–53.

Newsom-Davis, J. and Weatherall, D. J. (1994) *Health Policy and Technological Innovation*. London, Chapman & Hall.

NHS Centre for Reviews and Dissemination (1995) 'Aspirin and myocardial infarction'. *Effectiveness Matters* **1**: 1.

Noddings, N. (1984) *Caring: A Feminine Approach to Ethics and Moral Education*. Berkeley, CA, University of California Press.

Nolan, M. R. and Grant, G. (1989) 'Addressing the needs of informal carers: a neglected area of nursing practice'. *Journal of Advanced Nursing* **14**: 950–61.

Nolan, M., Grant, G. and Keady, J. (1996) *Understanding Family Care*. Buckingham, Open University Press.

Northway, R. (1997) 'Disability and oppression: some implications for nurses and nursing'. *Journal of Advanced Nursing* **26**: 736–43.

Norwich, H. S. and Senior, O. E. (1971) 'Determining nursing establishments'. *Nursing Times* **67**(5): 17–20.

Oakley, A. (1984) *The Captured Womb*. Oxford, Blackwell.

Oakley, A. (1996) *Man and Wife Richard and Kay Titmuss: My Parents' Early Years*. London, Flamingo.

Oakley, P. (1989) *Community Involvement in Health Development: An Examination of the Critical Issues*. Geneva, WHO.

Orem, D. E. (1991) *Nursing Concepts of Practice*. London, Mosby.

Osherson, S. and AmaraSingham, L. (1981) 'The machine metaphor in medicine', in Mishler, E. G. (ed.) *Social Contexts of Health Illness and Patient Care*. London, Cambridge University Press, pp. 218–49.

Øvretveit, J. (1993) *Co-ordinating Community Care: Multi-disciplinary Teams and Care Management*. Buckingham, Open University Press.

Parsons, T. (1979) 'Definitions of health and illness in the light of American values and social structure', in Jaco, E. G. (ed.) *Patients, Physicians and Illness*. New York, Free Press, pp. 120–44.

Pearson, A. (ed.) (1988) 'Primary nursing', in *Primary Nursing: Nursing in the Burford and Oxford Nursing Development Units*. London, Croom Helm, pp. 23–39.

Pearson, P., Procter, S., Allgar, V., Wilcockson, J., Lock, C., Spendiff, A., Davison, N., Taylor, G. and Foster, D. (1998) *Discharging Patients Effectively: Planning for Best Care*. Newcastle-upon-Tyne, University of Northumbria at Newcastle.

Peplau, H. E. (1993) *Interpersonal Relations in Nursing: a Conceptual Frame of Reference for Psychodynamic Nursing*. Basingstoke, Macmillan.

Pond, C. and Popay, J. (1983) 'Tackling inequalities at their source', in Glennerster, H. (ed.) *The Future of the Welfare State*. London, Heinemann, pp. 102–23.

Poole, J. (1998) 'A role change for auxiliaries'. *Nursing Times* **94**(44): 61.

Pott, E. (1992) 'Preface', in Kaplun, A. (ed.) *Health Promotion and Chronic Illness: Discovering a New Quality of Health.* Copenhagen, WHO Regional Office for Europe, pp. xi–xv.

Prescott, P. A. (1993) 'Nursing: an important component of hospital survival under a reformed health care system'. *Nursing Economics* **11**(4): 192–9.

Procter, S. (1989a) 'The functioning of nursing routines in the management of a transient workforce'. *Journal of Advanced Nursing* **14**: 180–9.

Procter, S. (1989b) A study of effects on the provision of nursing services of dependence on a learner nurse workforce to staff hospital wards. Unpublished PhD thesis, University of Northumbria, Newcastle-upon-Tyne.

Procter, S. (1995) 'Planning for continuity of carer in nursing'. *Journal of Nursing Management* **3**: 169–75.

Procter, S., Biott, C., Campbell, S., Edward, S., Redpath, N. and Moran, M. (1998) Preparation for the Developing Role of the Community Children's Nurse. Unpublished report. Newcastle-upon-Tyne, University of Northumbria at Newcastle.

Radwin, L. E. (1996) '"Knowing the patient": a review of research on an emerging concept'. *Journal of Advanced Nursing* **23**: 1142–6.

Rafferty, A. M. (1992) 'Nursing policy and the nationalization of nursing: the representation of "crisis" and the "crisis" of representation', in Robinson, J., Gray, A. and Elkan, R. (eds) *Policy Issues in Nursing.* Milton Keynes, Open University Press, pp. 68–83.

Read, S. (1994) 'Do formal controls always achieve control? The case of triage in accident and emergency departments'. *Health Services Management Research* **7**(1): 31–42.

Reder, P. and Lucey, C. (1995) 'Significant issues in the assessment of parenting', in Lucey, R. A. (ed.) *Assessment of Parenting: Psychiatric and Psychological Contributions.* London, Routledge, pp. 3–17.

Redfern, S. (1996) 'Individualised patient care: its meaning and practice in a general setting'. *NTResearch* **1**(1): 22–33.

Reed, J. (1992) 'Individualized patient care: some implications'. *Journal of Clinical Nursing* **1**: 7–12.

Reed, K. S. (1993) *Betty Neuman: the Neuman Systems Model.* London, Sage.

Rice, C., Roberts, H., Smith, S. J. and Bryce, C. (1992) 'It's like teaching your child to swim in a pool of alligators: lay voices and professional research on child accidents', in Popay, J. and Williams, G. (eds) *Researching the People's Health.* London, Routledge, pp. 115–33.

Riska, E. and Wegar, K. (eds) (1993) 'Women physicians: a new force in medicine?', in *Gender, Work and Medicine: Women and the Medical Division of Labour.* London, Sage, pp. 77–93.

Roach, S. M. (1985) 'A foundation for nursing ethics', in Carmi, A. and Schneider, S. (eds) *Nursing Law and Ethics.* Berlin, Springer-Verlag, pp. 170–7.

Robinson, J. (1989) 'Nursing in the future: a cause for concern', in Jolley, M. and Allan, P. (eds) *Current Issues in Nursing.* London, Chapman & Hall, pp. 151–78.

Robinson, J. and Elkan, R. (1997) 'Nursing up to and beyond the year 2000', in Salvage, J. and Heijnen, S. (eds) *Nursing in Europe: A Resource for Better Health.* Copenhagen, WHO Regional Office for Europe, pp. 127–44.

Rodgers, S. (1995) 'Accountability in primary nursing', in Watson, R. (ed.) *Accountability in Nursing Practice.* London, Chapman & Hall, pp. 70–91.

Rogers, M. (1980) 'Nursing: a science of unitary man', in Rheil, J. P. and Roy, C. (eds) *Conceptual Models for Nursing Practice*. New York, Appleton-Century-Crofts, pp. 329–37.

Rogers, M. E. (1970) *An Introduction to the Theoretical Basis of Nursing*. Philadelphia, F. A. Davis.

Roy, C. (1984) *Introduction to Nursing: an Adapatation Model*. London, Prentice Hall.

Royal College of Nursing (1992) *The Value of Nursing*. London, RCN.

Royal College of Nursing (1993) *Skill Mix: A Guide for RCN Members*. London, RCN.

Royal College of Physicians (1995) *Incontinence: Causes, Management and Provision of Services*. London, RCP .

Royal Commission on Long Term Care (1999) *With Respect to Old Age: Long Term Care Rights and Responsibilities*. London, Stationery Office.

Ruddick, S. (1989) *Maternal Thinking: Towards a Politics of Peace*. Boston, Beacon Press.

Runciman, P., Currie, C. T., Nicol, M., Green, L. and McKay, V. (1996) 'Discharge of elderly people from an accident and emergency department: evaluation of health visitor follow-up'. *Journal of Advanced Nursing* 24(4): 711–18.

Sackett, D. L. and Haynes, R. B. (1995) 'On the need for evidence-based medicine'. *Evidence-Based Medicine* 1(1): 5–6.

Salvage, J. and Heijnen, S. (1997) 'Nursing and midwifery in Europe', in Salvage, J. and Heijnen, S. (eds) *Nursing in Europe: A Resource for Better Health*. Copenhagen, WHO Regional Office for Europe, pp. 21–123.

Sanders, D. (1985) *The Struggle for Health: Medicine and the Politics of Underdevelopment*. London, Macmillan.

Schaffler, H.´(1992) 'Ayurveda: a long tradition of prevention', in Kaplun, A. (ed.) *Health Promotion and Chronic Illness: Discovering a New Quality of Life*. Copenhagen, WHO Regional Office for Europe, pp. 384–7.

Schnurre, M. (1992) 'Helping the patient sing his own song', in Kaplun A. (ed.) *Health Promotion and Chronic Illness: Discovering a New Quality of Life*. Copenhagen, WHO Regional Office for Europe, pp. 388–95.

Seedhouse, D. (1986) *Health: The Foundations for Achievement*. Chichester, Wiley.

Seedhouse, D. (1997) *Health Promotion Philosophy, Prejudice and Practice*. Chichester, Wiley.

Sharma, U. (1994) 'The equation of responsibility: complementary practitioners and their patients', in Budd, S. and Sharma, U. (eds) *The Healing Bond: The Patient–Practitioner Relationship and Therapeutic Responsibility*. London, Routledge, pp. 82–106.

Smedt, M. D. (1997) *Statistics in Focus: Population and Social Conditions*. Luxembourg, Eurostat.

Smith, P. (1992) *The Emotional Labour of Nursing*. Basingstoke, Macmillan.

Smith, P. and Agard, E. (1997) 'Care costs: towards a critical understanding of care', in Brykczynska, G. (ed.) *Caring: The Compassion and Wisdom of Nursing*. London, Arnold, pp. 180–204.

Sontag, S. (1978) *Illness as Metaphor*. Harmondsworth, Penguin.

Spaink, K. (1997) *The Chronically Ill: There Are no such People*. Empowerment of the Chronically Ill: A Challenge for Nursing. Amsterdam, paper presented at 2nd European Nursing Congress.

Spurgeon, P. (1993) *The New Face of the NHS*. Harlow, Longman.

Steering Committee Report (1996) *The Future Health Care Workforce*. Manchester, Health Services Management Unit, University of Manchester.

Stewart, M. J. and Tilden, V. P. (1995) 'The contributions of nursing science to social support'. *International Journal of Nursing Studies* **32**(6): 535–44.

Thomas, T. M., Plymat, K. R., Blannin J. and Meade, T. W. (1980) 'Prevalence of urinary incontinence'. *British Medical Journal* **281**: 1243–5.

Thorne, S. E. (1993) *Negotiating Health Care: The Social Context of Chronic Illness*. Thousand Oaks, CA, Sage.

Thorne, S. E. and Robinson, C. A. (1989) 'Guarded alliance: health care relationships in chronic illness'. *Journal of Nursing Scholarship* **21**: 153–7.

Tilden, V. P. and Weinert, C. (1987) 'Social support and the chronically ill individual'. *Nursing Clinics of North America* **22**(3): 613–19.

Titmuss, R. M. (1958) *Essays on the Welfare State*. London, Unwin.

Titmuss, R. M. (1970) *The Gift Relationship: From Human Blood to Social Policy*. London, Allen & Unwin.

Townsend, P. and Davidson, N. (eds) (1982) *Inequalities in Health*. Harmondsworth, Penguin.

Tschudin, V. (1997) 'The emotional cost of caring', in Brykczynska, G. (ed.) *Caring: The Compassion and Wisdom of Nursing*. London, Arnold, pp. 155–72.

Tudor-Hart, J. (1971) The inverse care law. *Lancet* (February): 405–12.

Twigg, J. (1989) 'Models of carers: how do social care agencies conceptualise their relationships with informal carers?' *Journal of Social Policy* **18**(1): 53–66.

Twigg, J. and Atkin, K. (1994) *Carers Perceived Policy and Practice in Informal Care*. Buckingham, Open University Press.

Twinn, S. and Cowley, S. (1992) *The Principles of Health Visiting: A Re-examination*. London, Health Visiting Association.

United Kingdom Central Council for Nursing, Midwifery and Health Visiting (1986) *Project 2000: A New Preparation for Practice*. London, UKCC.

United Kingdom Central Council for Nursing, Midwifery and Health Visiting (1992) *The Scope of Professional Practice: A UKCC Position Statement*. London, UKCC.

US Congress Office of Technology Assessment (1995) *Hospital Financing in Seven Countries*. Washington, DC, US Government Printing Office.

van den Bos, G. A. M. (1997) *Comprehensive Care for the Chronically Ill: Challenges for European Countries*. Empowerment of the Chronically Ill: A Challenge for Nursing. Amsterdam, paper presented at 2nd European Nursing Congress.

Walby, S., Greenwall, J., Mackay, L. and Soothill, K. (1994) *Medicine and Nursing. Professions in a Changing Health Service*. London, Sage.

Walford, D. (1994) 'The developed world', in Newson-Davis, J. and Weatherall, D. J. (eds) *Health Policy and Technological Innovation*. London, Chapman & Hall, pp. 3–26.

Ward, A. and McMahon, L. (1998) *Intuition is not Enough. Matching Learning with Practice in Therapeutic Childcare*. London, Routledge.

Warner, M., Longley, M., Gould, E. and Picek, E. (1998) *Healthcare Futures 2010*. London, UKCC/Education Commission.

Wass, A. (1994) *Promoting Health: The Primary Health Care Approach*. London, W. B. Saunders/Baillière Tindall.

Watson, J. (1985) *Nursing: Human Science and Human Care*. Norwalk, CT, Appleton-Century-Crofts.

Watson, W. (1998) 'Risk and coping in diabetes', in Heyman, B. (ed.) *Risk, Health and Health Care*. London, Arnold, pp. 187–98.

Whelan, J. (1998) *Leaving No Mans Land: Vision, Risk and the Eldonians*. Healthy Living Centre Conference, Gateshead.

Whitbeck, C. (1984) 'A different reality: feminist oncology', in Gould, C. C. (ed.) *Beyond Domination: New Perspectives on Women and Philosophy*. Totowa, NJ, Rowman & Allanheld, pp. 64–88.

White, R. (1985) 'Political regulators in British nursing', in White, R. (ed.) *Political Issues in Nursing: Past, Present and Future*. Chichester, Wiley, pp. 19–43.

Williams, G. (1986) *Save the Babies*. World Health Forum.

Winnicott, D. W. (1960) 'The theory of parent–infant relationship'. *International Journal of Psycho-Analysis* **41**: 585–95.

Workman, B. A. (1996) 'An investigation into how the health care assistants perceive their role as "support workers" to the qualified staff'. *Journal of Advanced Nursing* **23**: 612–19.

World Health Organization (1978) *Primary Health Care: A Report on the Conference on Primary Care (Alma Ata)*. Geneva, WHO.

World Health Organization (1986) *The Ottawa Charter for Health Promotion*. Ottawa, Canadian Public Health Association, Health and Welfare Canada.

World Health Organization (1997a) *The World Health Report 1997: Conquering Suffering, Enriching Humanity*. Geneva, WHO.

World Health Organization (1997b) *European Health Care Reform: Analysis of Current Strategies*. Copenhagen, WHO.

Yarnell, J. W. G., Voyle, G. J., Richards, C. J. and Stephenson, T. P. (1981) 'Prevalence and severity of urinary incontinence in women'. *Journal of Epidemiology and Community Health* **35**: 71–4.

Index

Page numbers printed in **bold** type refer to figures and in those *italic* to tables